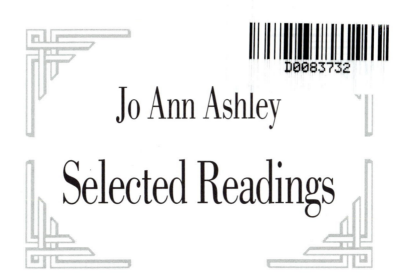

Jo Ann Ashley

Selected Readings

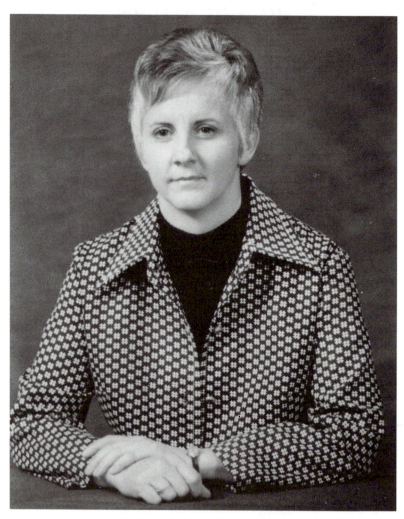

Jo Ann Ashley, 1939–1980

Jo Ann Ashley
Selected Readings

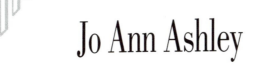

EDITED BY
KAREN ANNE WOLF, PhD, RN, CS

8-21-00
$ 33.95

NLN Press • New York
Pub. No. 15-6835

p. 23. "Reproduced from Dr. Jo Ann Ashley, "This I Believe, About Power in Nursing," *Nursing Outlook*, 1973, Vol. 21, pp. 637–641, with permission from Mosby-Year Book, Inc."

p. 103. © Texas Nurses Association 1976. Reprinted with permission from *TEXAS NURSING*, Vol. 50, No. 7, August 1976.

p. 157. Reprinted with permission of the MGH Institute of Health Professions. *American Journal of Nursing*, Volume 75 (no. 9), pp. 1465–1467.

Copyright © 1997
National League for Nursing
350 Hudson Street, New York, NY 10014

The views expressed in this book reflect those of the authors and do not necessarily reflect the official views of the National League for Nursing.

Library of Congress Cataloging-in-Publication Data

Jo Ann Ashley : selected readings / Karen Wolf, editor.
        p.   cm.
    "Pub. no. 15-6835."
    Includes bibliographical references and index.
    ISBN 0-88737-683-5
    1. Nursing—Social aspects. 2. Nursing—Political aspects.
3. Nursing—History. I. Ashley, Jo Ann, 1939–   II. Wolf,
Karen.
    [DNLM: 1. Ashley, Jo Ann, 1939–   2. Nursing—collected works.
WY 16 J62 1997]
RT86.5.J63   1997
610.73—dc21
                                                            96-49625
                                                            CIP

This book was set in Bodoni Book by Publications Development Company, Crockett, Texas. The editor and designer was Allan Graubard. The printer was Book Crafters. The cover was designed by Lauren Stevens.

Printed in the United States of America.

FOREWORD

*E*very movement for social, moral, or political change has its equivalent to the 6th-century BC Biblical Jeremiah—a prophet who cries out dire warnings about the need for reform in tough words and angry tones to a populace that cannot or will not hear. In many ways, Jo Ann Ashley became nursing's Jeremiah in the 1970s. While she did not brandish a staff nor rend her clothing, she did issue her uncompromising admonitions about why the failure to heed the consequences of nursing's historical suppression meant disaster for contemporary nursing practice and healthcare reform.

For many in nursing, particularly those in leadership or administration, the harshness of her historical vision made it impossible for them to understand or accept her message. But for thousands of others, especially those who read her 1976 book, *Hospitals, Paternalism and the Role of the Nurse*,[1] this Jeremiah was more like Moses. Her voice and visions made a direct connection to their own experiences and did so in a language few in nursing had felt it was possible to utter publicly.

As a feminist historian, health policy analyst (and non-nurse), I first encountered Ashley's writing in 1976 when I was a graduate student, working on a history of the development of American nursing.[2] While we both shared an understanding of the class, race, and gender oppression within nursing, our approach to the same primary historical sources was different.

In her book, Ashley tried to answer the question, "Why have nurses had so little influence on hospital management?" Ashley found the answer to this question in the paternalism of hospitals and physicians, the victimization of nurses through the apprenticeship system, and the failures of the nursing leadership to challenge the hierarchies of hospital/doctor/nurse. In often vituperative and angry words, not untypical of someone who feels they have been betrayed, Ashley's analysis sought to work out the relationships among the male chauvinism of doctors, the capitalist nature of American healthcare delivery, and the cultural devaluation of women's work. In delivering her attack upon these structures of oppression, Ashley came to see nurses primarily as victims, the equivalent of a powerless working class that emerged in much of Marx's writing on 19th-century workers and in some early feminist historical scholarship.

When I reviewed her book, I was critical of her use of the historical materials and her inability to see nurses as anything other than victims. What I missed as an historian was the need for a more complex analytic frame, a better understanding of the divisions within nursing itself, and a clearer analysis of the forms of resistance and political reforms that nurses *did* find possible.[3]

But as a non-nurse and an historian eager to have a sophisticated scholarly apparatus to explain nursing's history, I did not understand the importance of Ashley's historical message to many nurses. I did not fully appreciate how much she, and her mentor Theresa Christy, were laboring outside the supports in women's history that I could obtain. I shared Ashley's political concerns but had not experienced the same form of oppression she railed so strongly against. I had the privilege of being able to look at nursing from the outside. Ashley did not.

For many on the inside of nursing, Ashley's voice was prophetic and a wake-up call. It was the first time for a whole generation that the oppression of training, the expectation of second-class citizenship in the hospital, and the failure to hear the voices of caring nurses were named and denounced. As I spoke about Ashley's book to nursing audiences, I heard again and again that her book had helped them make sense of their own experiences, gave words to their own inchoate anger, explained why they were ignored and unappreciated in the hospital hierarchies.

Ashley's work, now from the perspective of twenty years of feminist scholarship on nursing history both by nurses who are historians and non-nurse historians of women's lives, must be seen as a necessary first step. Ashley's passion and anger were prophetic. It was necessary to speak in such tones just to be heard, to break through the socialization and *omerta*, or code of silence, that surrounded nursing. For many nurses, her anger made it possible for them to think about the feminist critiques of healthcare and nursing, to question the authority of physicians and hospital managements, to find a way to explain their experiences. Ashley's work thus provided a first contemporary feminist attempt to understand and critique nursing's past. Her words, as with much early feminist scholarship and writing, made political what had appeared before as only personal.

Others of us could build on what Ashley had done. We could find a different language to understand the nursing experience in more complex ways precisely because Ashley had opened up the questions. Twenty years later as an historian of the nursing experience, I still have concerns about her use of evidence and her portrait of nurses as merely victims. But as a women's studies scholar and feminist healthcare reform activist, I deeply understand her anger and admire her willingness literally to give her life to make a change in nursing. That we have gone on to use her work for nursing and healthcare reform is a tribute to her vision. Her efforts were of critical importance for nurses and many of us who do care passionately about what happens to American healthcare.

This collection of Ashley's writings, including her poetry, analysis of power, criticisms of nursing's rituals, and historical scholarship round out her vision that is only glimpsed in her previous book. Jeremiah's warnings may not have been heeded by the Israelites, but in the face of the dire condition of American healthcare, Ashley's should not be ignored.

Susan M. Reverby, PhD
Professor of Women's Studies
Wellesley College, Massachusetts

REFERENCES

1. Ashley, J. A. (1976). *Hospitals, paternalism, and the role of the nurse.* New York: Teachers College Press.

2. This work eventually became *Ordered to care: The dilemma of American nursing.* New York: Cambridge University Press, 1986.

3. See Susan Reverby, review of *Hospitals, paternalism and the role of the nurse* by Jo Ann Ashley in *Social Science and Medicine, 11* (April 1977): 443.

PREFACE

To know my sister, Jo Ann Ashley, was to know a scholar, a poet, a philosopher, a nurse, a historian, a teacher, a writer, an orator, and a social critic. These entities were interconnected, and each is reflected in her complete body of writings.

Born to parents who taught their children the value of truth, honesty, compassion, responsibility, and integrity, Jo Ann had an enormous intellect that enabled her to define and articulate the meaning of these and other values and to incorporate them into her personal philosophical foundation. Even as a teenager, she expressed her philosophical thoughts in the form of poetry. These early writings are interconnected with the totality of her adult philosophy wherein she expresses her basic premise that life is worthy of one's best Self. These early writings foretold her future as a historian and predicted how strongly and poignantly she would speak out about the injustices in society. Portions of one poem are a summation:

> . . . Give to Life the best you have . . .
> . . . Give to this an ardent Self . . . .
>   A Sincerity that will not fade
>   And life will have been a thing you made
>   As you called a spade a spade.

Jo Ann, the philosopher, was a seeker of truth, a thinker, and a scholar of the writings of philosophers and social critics—ancient, classical, and contemporary. Her belief that freedom of thought brought freedom of being inspired her to urge nurses and all women to recognize that "political freedom is basically intellectual freedom: the freedom to do one's own thinking." She cautioned that as long as individuals were in the position of being dependent on others for doing their thinking, they would be "kept powerless and often used to meet the ends of other people's desires."

Jo Ann, the poet, viewed poetic language as an excellent avenue for expressing symbolic meaning. She expressed her innermost thoughts concerning nurses, healthcare, society, power, and what it means to be human, in the form of poetic expression. She rarely included her poetry in presentations, but on one occasion of sharing her poetry, she stated, "My main concerns in life are truth, justice, and the beauty of health in human life. Poetry deals with a truth that can sometimes touch the human heart giving birth to new ideas, new emotions, new energies, and new growth." She used poetic expression as a means of chronicling her journey through life, as well as a means of expressing freedom of thought. Her poems, speeches, and articles were interconnected.

Jo Ann, the teacher, loved teaching. She inspired her students to become independent thinkers and encouraged them to cultivate inner courage in order to gain the power and freedom needed to rehumanize society. She taught them how to look into themselves and find the power that was within them.

Jo Ann, the nurse, found, through her own life experiences, the true meaning of how social thought and social order could perpetuate oppression, abuse, exploitation, and repression. Having had firsthand experience, she was able to describe, in the proper context, these injustices done to individual living human beings. Her compassion and sensitivity enabled her to communicate, in relevant, truthful, descriptive language, the true reality of nursing's history.

Jo Ann, the nurse historian, went to the root of nursing's history to analyze the problems facing nurses and women in society. She attempted to find answers to society's devaluation of the worth of nurses as vital participants in providing healthcare. She examined the history of social thought about women, giving special emphasis to political, economic, social, and cultural forces shaping the lives of nurses, and how these forces influenced nurses' self-image, public image, and actions. She went to the primary sources, recounting in their own words the attitudes of nurses and women in general. She named the oppressors, identified the injustices, and examined the effects these injustices had on nurses. Her theory was: "Oppression is a form of deception in which one human being is led to believe [he or she exists] to meet the needs of another human being or institution."

Jo Ann, the philosopher and social critic, could intellectualize how this social view of women, and the deceptive use of altruistic language, was used as a tool to weaken and to conquer the human spirit of nurses, and to make them feel powerless. This deception created and perpetuated social and professional fragmentation for nurses as individuals and as a group. She understood the writings of other social critics concerning this social and psychological phenomenon of how "the masses of people, who are under the hypnotic influence of those who wish to control them, grow accustomed to being told they cannot trust in their own reason, but must be guided by what others tell them." Jo Ann defined this behavior as "adhesion to the oppressor." The oppressed become so closely allied with those who dominate and control them that they cannot achieve enough distance to objectively evaluate themselves as beings separate from their oppressors. Therefore, their lack of insight, of understanding, and of objectivity about the reality of their situation prevents them from seeking to truly break away from the circumstances that oppress them.

She understood how nurses were being used as tools of oppression in their role as agents and as managers of policies and actions implemented to perpetuate hate and distrust among their peers. This distrust, in turn, maintained fragmentation.

Jo Ann urged nurses to recognize and see through the myths, illusions, and deceptions that have strengthened the chains binding them to the past. She stressed to nurses: "The bigotry among nurses and the hatred they commonly share toward one another is an outgrowth of oppression, stupidity, and unconscious motivations having deep roots within society, and within the institutions where nurses are educated and where they work."

Preface

Jo Ann's educational emphasis in social thought, her prophetic wisdom, and her ability to envision a future in which nurses would have freedom to do their own thinking and to choose their own directions and actions, gave her the courage to boldly and poignantly speak out about the injustices against nurses. Her strength and courage earned her the label "angry woman," from critics who could not get past their own structures of mind, instilled through myths and deceptions. Jo Ann remained undaunted in her examination of realities and her search for truths within society and in the healthcare system.

Wanting to make Jo Ann's writing accessible to scholars, historians, and other readers, our mother has generously donated Jo Ann's writings and research materials to The Center for The Study of The History of Nursing, University of Pennsylvania School of Nursing, Philadelphia, Pennsylvania. It is our hope that the historians of the present and the future will give Jo Ann the recognition and respect she deserves for her role in exposing society's evils against nurses and all women.

Our mother, Jo Ann's sisters, brother, and I express our appreciation and gratitude to Dr. Karen Wolf for her continued interest in Jo Ann's valuable contribution to nursing, and for the compilation of Jo Ann's selected works. We express our appreciation and thanks to Dr. Patricia Moccia, Chief Executive Officer, National League for Nursing, and Mr. Allan Graubard, Director, National League for Nursing Press, for the publication of this book.

Jo Ann's speeches and writings are as timely today as they were when she spoke and wrote them. Guided by her philosophy that intellectual freedom of thought gives direction to action, Jo Ann usually prefaced her speeches by saying, "I ask you to seriously *think* about what I say, raise questions about it, have *open* discussions with groups of your classmates [and] colleagues about it. . . . I want you to take your thoughts home with you, to work with you; think about them as you interact with classmates or other professionals. Urge others to help you examine the issues involved and their importance for healthcare in this nation." Jo Ann, the thinker, the philosopher, the teacher, the orator, the poet, and the writer would say the same words today.

We remain saddened by our loss, but we find comfort in knowing that, through her writings, Jo Ann will live as her words empower others to freedom of thought and action. Her writings will continue to be that needed voice for change. The reading of her *own* words will show her complex understanding of nursing's historical and present dilemmas. Her own words are important sources for a complete understanding of her legacy to nursing and society.

Edith Ashley Shinbach, RN

About the Editor

Karen Anne Wolf, PhD, RN, CS, is on the faculty of the Graduate Program in Nursing at the MGH Institute of Health Professions in Boston and maintains a practice at the Cambridge Senior Health Center. A diploma graduate from the Johns Hopkins Hospital School of Nursing, she received her BSN and MS in Community Health Nursing from Boston University, a post masters Certificate in Adult Health from the University of Massachusetts/Worcester, and doctorate in Sociology from Brandeis University. Dr. Wolf has written and spoken widely on the topics of politics and nursing, community health, and women's health and aging. She has served as a consultant to a variety of media projects and has been active with groups such as Nurses Now, Nurses for Progressive Social Change, and Nurses for National Health Care. In her spare time, she makes apple butter and shoofly pie with her family.

ACKNOWLEDGMENTS

Some fifteen years ago, I expressed the desire to see Dr. Ashley's papers preserved for future generations of nurses. I am grateful that Dr. Ashley's family has held to this same desire. I thank Dr. Ashley's mother, Mrs. Jewel Ashley, for granting me the privilege to compile this volume. Since her death, Dr. Ashley's sister, Edith Shinbach, has preserved and organized the collection with tremendous care. In addition, she has provided enthusiasm and archival assistance for this project. I thank the entire Ashley family for their support and encouragement. Despite the renewed sense of grief and loss, the family has rallied to celebrate Jo Ann's life and work.

This project was made possible by the effort of the National League for Nursing Press. I am indebted to Dr. Patricia Moccia, NLN CEO, and Allan Graubard, Director of NLN Press, for their commitment to this project. Over the years I have benefitted from the critical insights and support from nursing colleagues and feminists. I wish to remember Nurses for Progressive Social Change, Nurses Now, DSA Nurses, Cassandra, Nurses Network, the Boston Women's Health Book Collective, and the Brandeis University Sociology Department for their role in sustaining the belief in feminism and a vision of social change.

This project has been supported by a sabbatical leave from the Graduate Program in Nursing at the MGH Institute of Health Professions. In addition, I benefited from the research assistance of Heather Ackerman and secretarial expertise of Valarie Grande. My students and patients, past present and future have fueled this work, as did my encounters with the former colleagues and students of Dr. Ashley.

Last but not least, I wish to thank my extended Wolf-Oberholtzer family for encouraging my efforts, tolerating my absorption, and sharing in the juggling of childcare and career.

Dr. Ashley's papers have recently been donated to the University of Pennsylvania Nursing Archives in Philadelphia. As part of the Nursing History Archives, her papers will continue to inspire future generations to reflect on the historic struggles of nurses and the potential for health promoting social change.

KAREN ANNE WOLF

CONTENTS

Contents

INTRODUCTION

Problems surrounding the American healthcare system derived from a process of historical development that has its roots in changes and events that occurred in the early part of the century. Today's concerns have been the concerns of the past as well: there are no controls on costs or quality in hospitals; administrators and physicians remain more concerned about their own interests than those of their patients; hospitals and doctors are accused of profiteering in the health business at the expense of the public good. Moreover, there is no national health policy nor any efforts toward national planning for health preservation; provisions for quality and social economy have either been ignored or defeated largely by private interest groups, of which the American Medical Association is a prime example. Health has remained a private matter and yet has to become a public responsibility. (Ashley, 1976 pp. 123–124)

Voices from the past echo into the future, illuminating the reasons for current crises and guiding us in our quest for change. This collection of papers by the late Dr. Jo Ann Ashley, feminist historian, nursing activist and educator, record her powerful voice and her call for social change. Speaking out for the empowerment of nurses and the creation of a more humane healthcare system, her message and inspiration remain relevant as we confront a continuing crisis in healthcare.

By definition, a crisis lasting more than twenty years is not a crisis. Yet the American healthcare system has been labeled as in crisis since the early 1970s. During this decade, concern about healthcare inflation, poor quality of care, and the pursuit of National Health Insurance has dominated the debates.

In the ensuing twenty years, healthcare costs have mounted while access to care has declined. Despite the rise in uninsured to more than 40 million people and the growing evidence of declining health status in the United States, large scale reform is unlikely to occur soon.

The power and politics of healthcare addressed by Dr. Ashley continue to be mired in patriarchal and profit-making structures. Major stakeholders in the healthcare industry—insurers, hospitals, and physician groups such as the American Medical Association—have been successful at blocking major reforms. While the movement for healthcare reform may have failed in the short term, competitive pressures and regulatory changes by government are reshaping the healthcare system. The escalation of healthcare costs has fueled the development of large networks of managed care services. Insurance companies and the federal government are aligned in their efforts to cut costs by forcing hospitals and providers to compete.

As a result, increasing competition has left providers and patients whirling in the wake of mergers and marketing. Faced with the new language of HMOs, PPOs, networks, and alliances, the public is confused and frustrated.

Who will advocate for the public? Dr. Ashley posed this question some twenty years ago. Her condemnation of medical paternalism, the depersonalizing healthcare experience, and the social injustices that create illness and despair was harsh and direct. She held the hope that nurses could free themselves from their long-standing oppression as professionals and become a force for the re-humanization of healthcare.

Along with other healthcare providers as well, nurses today find themselves in a contradictory position. Struggling to achieve professional autonomy in an increasingly bureaucratic maze of care, providers become even more entrenched in maintaining the system as it is. Advocacy for change has taken a back seat to entrepreneurism. Self-interest and survivalism have become a first priority. As the healthcare system reverses incentives on healthcare spending, healthcare providers are squeezed between guidelines for care and constraints on allowable costs. Healthcare providers are also often told to adapt to the current system or to opt out.

Nonetheless, primary care expansion is ending the dominance of specialty care by physicians. While a much needed development, the end of such physician dominance is offset by reductions in care giving generally. The speed-up in outpatient care, reduction in hospital stays, and stringent limits to home care, rehabilitation, and mental health services compromises health restoration. Pressures to reduce healthcare costs have hit the healthcare labor force hard, forcing downsizing of hospitals and fueling competition between primary care providers and specialists.

Nurses, long the backbone of the healthcare system, are also under siege by the growing trend of hospital downsizing. While community care rhetoric increases, pubic health program funding decreases, with the community labor market expansion slow to compensate for the loss of career opportunities, benefits, and wages of the still primary hospital labor sector.

In regard to nurse practitioners specifically, the shift to a primary care focus has generated new tensions between them and physicians. More nurses are returning for advanced practice education as nurse practitioners while at the same time medical schools and residency are retooling for primary care. Competition begins with educational programs as each discipline vies for practice sites for training. The drive to attract patients and reimbursement is mounting as providers compete to fill patient volume quotas.

Nurse practitioners have also, and unfortunately, not been able to overcome the underlying structural barriers of patriarchal medicine. Collaboration with physician colleagues is hard to achieve as institutional pressure and incentives give precedence to medicine. Despite their twenty-year history of care to underserved populations and of collaborative practice, advanced practice nurses of many sorts find that they are usually invisible as policy deliberation and contract negotiation between insurers and providers proceeds.

Amidst this continuing crisis, it is the American public that suffers most. We are challenged to look critically at our situation. Many of the questions raised by Dr. Ashley in this volume continue to be the subject of debate:

- Is the healthcare system a threat to the health of the public; or can you reshape a system that is fundamentally flawed by its profit making drive and patriarchal structure?
- What effect does the profit motive in healthcare have on the outcomes of care? Does the profit motive contribute to the erosion of good healthcare or the perpetuation of inadequate healthcare?
- Can we have an equitable and humane healthcare system if there is a failure to provide access to nursing as well as to medical care?
- How do stakeholders group such as medicine, hospitals, and insurers remain so powerful while other groups such as nurses struggle to be heard?
- Consider the power of women to ban together to end oppression in our social institutions such as healthcare, schools, industry, or government. If providers such as nurses were to gain greater power, would we use it to move beyond self-interest?
- Can the American public muster the moral and political will to create social change for a health promoting healthcare system?

By reviewing our past, we can identify patterns of social behaviors, and the underlying structures that give rise to our current crisis. Dr. Ashley observed that the crisis in healthcare reflects not only our society's lack of political will, but also a devaluing of human caring.

The many facets of nursing history serve to mirror our societal tensions and conflict. According to Dr. Ashley, the oppression and economic exploitation of nursing and the struggle of nurses to unite as a group to advance their interests reflect the power of capitalist patriarchy. In her 1976 book *Hospitals, Paternalism and the Role of the Nurse*, Dr. Ashley urged that:

> Given recent and current criticisms of poor quality in healthcare, the public would do well to turn more of its attention to developments in nursing, and to the problems with which this group has to contend. For a century, defects in nursing service have provided an index to general defects in America's healthcare system. (Ashley, 1976, p. 132)

In the twenty years since the publication of *Hospitals, Paternalism and the Role of the Nurse*, the perpetuation of patriarchal systems and economic exploitation continues to undermine the development of a health promoting healthcare system. The contradictions posed by a profit-oriented healthcare nonsystem tears at the ethos of caring as nurses find themselves struggling for professional and personal survival. While the paternalism of hospital controls may be obscured by the transformation of healthcare systems, new forms of patriarchy and oppression are emerging under the competitive din of market competition and managed care.

Nursing, empowered in the late 1970s to 1980s by professional gains in education, practice, and legislation, is once again fearing a loss of power. With cost-cutting efforts targeting nursing budgets, the advances of the 1980s are threatened by institutional take backs. Overproduction of the nursing labor supply by nursing education programs also promises to add to nursing's woes. Without a change in the current labor trajectory, depressed wages, underemployment, and massive unemployment can become inevitable. Although such unemployment would differ substantially from the experience of the 1930s, the current willingness of nursing education, for example, to sustain the downward labor trajectory by overproduction should be of great concern. Is nursing the passive victim here or is nursing merely demonstrating more sophisticated means of exploitation by which it continues to integrate and carry out the will of its oppressors?

Some twenty years after Jo Ann Ashley spoke out on the state of healthcare, the urgency for fundamental change mounts. Viewed by Dr. Ashley as a major resource for social activism and caring, nurses must reclaim their moral courage and political power.

This selection of papers and poems by Dr. Jo Ann Ashley is intended to inspire readers to continue to challenge actively for change. Her work provides a link from the struggles and gains of the past to our potential to help shape the future. Her work, her voice, and her belief in our power to act responsibly helped to lay the foundation for nursing empowerment. The crisis we face in healthcare today provides an opportunity to create new alliances for the re-humanization of healthcare. Passionate concern for the future of nursing, the future of healthcare, and the future of human caring is critical as we move toward the next millennium.

ABOUT THE LIFE AND WORK OF DR. ASHLEY

When Dr. Jo Ann Ashley died of breast cancer at the young age of 41 in 1980, her death stunned a generation of nurses who felt the power of her leadership and nursing advocacy. The loss of her passionate voice and leadership in the empowerment of nursing and the improvement of healthcare was felt across the United States. In memorium, it was written that:

> Dr. Ashley's fiery indictment of the medical domination of nursing stirred the collective consciousness of nurses around the world. Dr. Ashley repeatedly called upon nurses to recognize the intentional fragmentation of the nursing profession and to unite. (Wolf, 1981)

Her short life was rich in professional accomplishments made possible through the loving support of family and friends. A dedicated nurse educator, she was drawn to social activism and feminism through her study of nursing history. The social climate of the 1960s and early 1970s created a powerful base for her developing social criticism. In her efforts to attain education beyond the basic nursing diploma, she had first-hand experience with the barriers that women faced. Like most nurses of this period, she chose nursing out of a restricted field of career opportunities. Unlike most nurses of her day, however, she placed tremendous value on intellectual pursuit and held on to her dream for further education.

Born in rural Kentucky, Jo Ann Ashley typified a generation of rural women who gained access to an affordable education through hospital-based diploma nursing programs. She loved Kentucky and was most comfortable in the rolling hills surrounding the small family farm in Sweeton. Walking across the fields provided her with the solitude to think and to write. Growing up in a large family of six children meant that there were few personal spaces and resources. Her family and teachers encouraged her natural abilities as a student and her desire to be a voracious reader and writer. During her childhood she began writing poetry as a means for personal reflection and she continued this throughout her life. She graduated first in her rural high school class.

Early in life she also developed a belief in her own abilities and a drive to further her education. She was one of four nurses in her family and attended her basic nursing education program with her older sister, Jane. Although she began her education at Western Kentucky College, she transferred to the Kentucky Baptist Hospital during her first year. Receiving her B.S. degree at Catherine Spaulding College, Jo Ann worked as a psychiatric staff nurse and as a nursing instructor in Kentucky.

In her early staff nurse experiences, she began to observe how little respect nurses were given for their intelligence and contribution to patient care. Her quest for further education was encouraged by colleagues and her family and made possible through the infusion of federal monies for graduate education that began in the late 1960s. When she decided to go on to graduate school, she set her sights on Teachers College at Columbia University. As the oldest graduate program in the country, Teachers College carried a strong reputation for leadership and intellectual rigor. Her acceptance into Teachers College thrust Jo Ann into the tumultuous world of New York City in the late 1960s.

Growing up in a rural community with a clearly defined social structure and traditional relations accentuated the social disparities and injustices that Jo Ann found in New York City. While she worked on her Masters in Psychiatric and Community Nursing and as a staff nurse in New York Veterans Administration Hospital, her questioning of the social order intensified. She began to see connections between the experiences of nurses, frustrated in their inability to provide quality care, and in the growing debate on humanizing healthcare. Nonetheless, while the "concentrated misery" of New York was of a greater magnitude than that of rural Kentucky, the underpinnings were the same. Her poetry captures the pain of this period:

> I saw old women and old men on the streets of
> New York City.
> They were dirty, unclean, and sick.
> I had the knowledge and hands that could have
> helped these old women,
> These old men.
> I am a nurse
>
> The old men and women I saw on the
> streets of New York City will die with
> Their fingernails dirty and uncut.
> They are not human.
> Is this not a shameful thing and
> A sad reflection upon our whole society?
> Only a Nurse politically free can help
> What ails our society.
>
> (From *What a Nurse Can See on the Streets of New York City*, J. A. Ashley)

Nursing was not immune to the social movements of the time for greater equality. The opportunities for education and a career in nursing mirrored that of society structured by long-standing assumptions about gender, race, and class. Dr. Ashley confronted many of these assumptions and myths as she worked to attain first her diploma and baccalaureate degree and later her graduate degrees. Her enjoyment and pursuit of scholarship also countered a then pervasive anti-intellectualism in nursing. As Dr. Ashley noted, hospital nursing education flourished because there were few alternatives. By the

1960s the barriers to collegiate education in nursing were just beginning to crumble. Nurses faced discriminatory double standards in education and practice. Widespread inequities in pay and limited opportunities for advancement forced many nurses out of the field. For Dr. Ashley, graduate education in nursing offered the best chance for a secure career path as a nursing educator and the opportunity to apply her intellectual abilities.

During the late 1960s and early 1970s, New York City was in turmoil. Student protests were common and students as a group contributed much to a burgeoning anti-war movement, women's movement, and movement for racial equality. As Jo Ann stayed on at Columbia Teachers College for doctoral studies, she too began to participate in social change movements. Her introduction to feminism and social activism had a profound effect on her thinking. While Dr. Ashley's original intention was to study philosophy, she found herself drawn more to the history of social thought. Her dissertation study was later revised and published by Teachers College Press as the groundbreaking *Hospitals, Paternalism and the Role of the Nurse.*

After the completion of her doctorate, she took a position as assistant professor at Pennsylvania State University. Just as she made her move to Pennsylvania, she returned to Kentucky for a diagnosis and treatment of her breast cancer. After a brief tenure at Penn, she moved on to Northern Illinois University in Chicago where she held the rank of Associate Professor. The period at Northern Illinois was her most productive, leading with more than three dozen presentations and a dozen publications. The themes of "power and politics" and the linking of nurses' rights to consumer rights in healthcare predominated. Her writings were grounded in her own experiences as she continued her commitment to nursing and feminist political action. She became a founding member of the Nurses' Coalition for Action in Politics (NCAP), the political action committee associated with the American Nurses Association (ANA), and was a member of the Illinois State Committee for Equal Rights for Women as a representative for the Nursing Association. She sought contact with feminist groups such as NOW and encouraged and corresponded with the group Nurses NOW.

In 1977, she was offered a position as a full professor and chair-personship at Texas Women's University. A major career advancement, she was excited by this opportunity to work with doctoral students. Unfortunately her arrival coincided with a major institutional turmoil at that university.

After a brief but tumultuous year, she took a position at Wright State University. She found renewed support under the leadership of Gertrude Torres and with feminist colleagues such as Peggy Chinn. Shortly after receiving her tenure as a full professor, the illusion of institutional peace was shattered again by crisis. The university administration proposed to establish a second nursing education program outside the administration of the School of Nursing and under the authority of the Medical School as a proposed solution to "community," that is, local hospitals', needs. The implication here was clear: the School of Nursing was unresponsive and lacking in quality clinical experience. Ironically, the School of Nursing had recently received full accreditation from the National League for Nursing with mention of their innovative educational program. After finding the university administration unwilling to reverse their decision, the dean and many of the nursing faculty resigned. Committed to the principle of nursing faculty having control over their own curriculum, Dr. Ashley joined the departing ranks. The experience reverberated as another chapter in her study of nursing and paternalism.

There is no doubt, too, that Jo Ann's departure came at great personal cost. Dr. Ashley was experiencing the progression of her cancer and the pleading of her family to avoid the strain of another move. Within six months of starting her new position at West Virginia University, she recognized that her death was imminent. She returned to Kentucky one last time for the funeral of her father and within two months stopped struggling against the cancer and died.

Diagnosed with breast cancer in her thirties, she maintained a vigorous life of teaching, research, writing, and political action. Her own personal struggles with cancer were not to be publicly acknowledged. Dr. Ashley was well aware of the stigma attached to "cancer," and she feared that her words and work would be delegitimated if her illness were publicly known. As her disease progressed from the early 1970s to the latter part of the decade, her work becomes more reflective of the greater social challenges taking place around her. As poet Audre Lorde wrote of her experience with breast cancer in *The Cancer Journals* (1980):

> Living a self-conscious life, under the pressure of time I work with the consciousness of death at my shoulder, not constantly, but often enough to leave a mark upon all my life's decisions and actions. And it does not matter whether this death comes next week or thirty years from now; this self-consciousness gives my life another breadth. It helps shape the strength of my vision and my purpose, the depth of my appreciation of living. (p. 16)

Dr. Ashley's commitment to speaking out about the injustices of healthcare and the oppression of nurses placed her in peril. She was denounced for her open criticism of medicine and for her alliance with feminism. Similarly, Audre Lorde speaks of the urgency of her own efforts as a social critic: "I have come to believe over and over again that what is most important to me must be spoken, made verbal and shared, even at the risk of having been bruised or misunderstood" (1980, p. 19).

Throughout her life, Dr. Ashley had a great appreciation for words, and language became her most powerful tool. She drew on vivid imagery, occasionally polemical, but powerfully delivered with the punch of a sermon. Her speeches were often dismissed by the members of the medical profession and elite nursing colleagues as "mere anger." She greeted this dismissal with a calm resignation. She understood only too well that the label of "angry" was commonly applied to other feminists writers of past and present. She was in good company with such writers as Virgina Woolf, who was condemned as angry, shrill, or strident for essays such as "The Three Guineas" (Barrett, 1979). Carolyn Heilbrun points out the dismissive intent of such labeling, saying, "To denounce women for shrillness and stridency is another way of denying them any right to power"(1988, p. 16).

Through the decade of the 1970s, Dr. Ashley's evolving feminist analysis came to include a variety of liberal, radical, and socialist perspectives. Consistent throughout her writings was her attempt to connect the personal struggles of nurses to the larger political economy of healthcare. She received many letters from nurses and the public in response to her presentations or media interviews, telling her of their personal struggles. Frequently she would share their stories in her presentations, recognizing that her public voice was a way to make visible their hidden suffering.

Jo Ann Ashley was a forceful advocate for social change and nursing activism. Beginning in the early 1970s, she provided a decade of charismatic leadership grounded in feminist principles. Her commitment to advancing the interests of nurses was rooted in her belief that this would be beneficial to the public. A critic of self-interested politics, Dr. Ashley spoke out against the perpetuation of forms of domination such as patriarchy and capitalist exploitation. Perhaps best known for her book, *Hospital, Paternalism and the Role of the Nurse*, Dr. Ashley was one of the rare nursing leaders of this century who was willing to speak out and to embrace feminism both in her scholarship and as a basis for social action. As Roberts and Group note in their book *Feminism and Nursing* (1992), like Lavinia Dock before her Ashley saw the perpetuation of patriarchy through legal and educational systems keenly exemplified by the development of hospital nursing in the United States. The subordination of nursing to the interests of medicine and hospital administration was achieved through structural and ideological oppression. The good nurse was one who best served the interest of the physician and the hospital. Ashley also argued here that nursing leadership especially lacked the following of staff nurses. Instead, the power of nursing leadership was vested in its service to medicine. According to Ashley, the true power of nursing could only be realized when nurses would come to nurture one another and unite.

A prolific writer and highly sought after public speaker, she gave over 75 presentations and interviews from 1975 to 1980. As Dr. Ashley described her own work, writing in November 1977:

I have thought long and hard about the image of nursing . . . about the meaning of power and how nurses can use their power and its use in fostering the work of nursing. I have fought long and hard for the rights of nurses attempting in my writings to provide new insights to clarify our situation and the symptoms of social illness that plague every step we take. (Ashley, 1977)

Her desire to advocate for the fuller recognition of nursing's potential to help society, and her sense of urgency, propelled her to adopt a demanding pace on the lecture circuit. She frequently gave two or more presentations a month to diverse audiences of healthcare providers, women's groups, and the public. She drew on current events with vivid scenarios from nursing practice to capture the attention of her audience.

With forceful, direct language, she sought to break the passivity of nurses, viewing it as simply another manifestation of false consciousness. Directed at the "staff nurse on the wards" much like "the man in the streets," many of her presentations had a folksy quality as well. Despite the high value she placed on intellectual development and critical thinking, Dr. Ashley recognized the inherent divisiveness of intellectual elitism. She sought to have her message heard, speaking passionately, imbuing her speeches with poignant examples of social injustices from the lives of nurses and the public.

While she spoke to her audiences about the legacy of nursing history, she pushed nurses, other healthcare providers, and the public to take up political action. She admonished others to ground their power and politics in the ethos of caring. For Dr. Ashley, the power and politics of nursing was inherently the issue of the power and politics of women.

Educated as a historian and educator, Dr. Ashley was widely regarded as an influential nursing scholar and teacher. In her work with graduate students, she was known to be challenging, inspiring, and intellectually rigorous. Foremost was her desire to enable her students to think critically and develop their own ideas and interpretations. She continued to teach in her practice area of community mental health as well as in theory, research, and healthcare politics.

I was introduced to her work by a feminist nurse consciousness raising group in the early 1970s with the reading of the article, "This

I Believe About Power and Nursing." In 1978, I also became involved with Dr. Ashley in the production of a film documentary "Nursing: the Politics of Caring in the mid-1970's" (Fanlight Films 1978). Working with filmmakers Joan Finck Sawyer and Timothy Sawyer to present a picture of the issues that were facing nurses in the mid 1970s, I urged the inclusion of Dr. Ashley, who agreed to travel to Boston for the filming in 1976 and for a meeting with the local Nurses NOW group. During the filming she spoke forcefully about the societal need for nursing care and the longstanding hospital and medical paternalism that served as a barrier. Over dinner, she stated with conviction that "the doctors are going to kill me!" I was unaware until years later the anguish she experienced around the diagnosis of her breast cancer. The diagnosis was delayed when her New York physician refused to take her concern over a breast lump as valid. She was finally diagnosed by a family physician in Kentucky who took seriously her concern and her family history of breast cancer. Despite her many moves, she continued to receive her cancer care in Kentucky, supported and cared for by her family.

Dr. Ashley opened the way to future generations of nurses to call into question the state of healthcare and to align with consumers to push for more patient-centered and humane healthcare as well as improved social conditions for health. She generated renewed interest in the history of nursing and helped to build the bridge between feminism and nursing. Some fifteen years after her death, women, including many nurses, are engaged in social activism around such health issues as national health reform, AIDS, violence prevention, and breast cancer awareness. As she approached the end of her life, she expressed the wish that her papers be published and the hope that the work she had begun would continue.

The papers and poems in this collection were selected to highlight Dr. Ashley's perspectives and to preserve the uniqueness of her "voice." While she wrote more than 70 papers during the decade preceding her death, many of her papers recapitulated similar themes and references. I have included selections which present a distinct perspective and have the potential to generate thoughtful debate.

Introduction

References

Ashley, J. A. (1974). *What a nurse can see on the streets of New York City* (unpublished poem, Ashley archives).

_____ . (1976). *Hospitals, paternalism and the role of the nurse.* New York: Teachers College Press.

_____ . (1977). "The image of nursing: Pride in power." Keynote address to the State Convention of the Massachusetts Nurses Association, Worcester, Massachusetts.

Barrett, M. (Ed.). (1980). *Virgina Woolf, Women and writing.* New York: Harcourt Brace & Company (A Harvest Book).

Heilbrun, C. (1988). *Writing a woman's life.* New York: Ballantine Books.

Lorde, A. (1980) *The cancer journals.* San Francisco: Aunt Lute Books.

Roberts, J. I., & Group, T. M. (1994). *Feminism and nursing, an historical perspective on power, status and political activism in the nursing profession.* Westport, CT: Praegar.

Wolf, K. A. (May 1981). A memorium to Dr. Jo Ann Ashley. The *Massachusetts Nurse.*

PART ONE

POWER AND POLITICS

*T*he 1990s movement for healthcare reform reflected a nursing activism unprecedented in past decades. A nursing coalition drafted a nursing agenda for healthcare reform, bringing together dozens of different nursing constituencies. Oppositional groups pressed for a National Healthcare System. The growing political power base in nursing and its current sophistication owe much to the groundwork laid by activist leaders such as Jo Ann Ashley. When she began her campaign to raise the consciousness of nurses to the realities of power and politics, Jo Ann Ashley frequently confronted apathy and avoidance. Politics carried a negative connotation and nurses felt powerless to bring about change. As American society faced the turmoil and social movements for equal rights for women and blacks, consumer rights, the women's health movement and others, some nurses began to press for change.

In the 1970s, concerns about power and politics in nursing and healthcare escalated. Nurses sought equality through governmental and workplace reforms. Dr. Jo Ann Ashley was at the forefront of the nursing politicalization effort, urging nurses to recognize, cultivate, and use their power effectively. In her travels across the country, she spoke out, urging nurses to refuse to be satisfied with the status quo, to avoid the oppression it brought with it. Reaching out to the diversity of nursing interests, she addressed issues from educational access and entry into practice to workplace conditions and unionism. Often at the middle of controversy, she was a risk taker who raised the issues despite the personal costs. She argued that the "oppression of the past" has not ended and that nursing continues to be subordinated to the interests of medicine and the hospital industry.

In her poem *Components of Power*, Dr. Ashley relates "the acquisition of the power demands a loss of innocence." To Ashley, this meant giving up the naive belief that the "handmaiden role to medicine" was a societal good. Rather, nursing must recognize that the continuing subordination of nursing to medicine and hospitals largely hindered public access to the mature potential of nursing practice. From the feminist perspective, the continuing subordination of nurses as women reflected the perpetuation of patriarchal beliefs that women are inherently evil, less intelligent, less capable, and need to be controlled and protected by men. Dr. Ashley also recognized the willingness of many nursing leaders to sacrifice other nurses to achieve or maintain their own power. She cautioned nurses to "beware of where you place your feet, if your freedom you have not obtained, you may end up following the very devil and never even know it." Her criticism of nursing complicity drew the wrath of some nursing elite, such as nursing administrators, and at the same time built a supportive following from rank and file nurses.

The papers selected for this section were written during the 1970s, and highlight Dr. Ashley's commitment to developing power and political potential in nursing. Many of the papers were efforts at consciousness raising through publication in mainstream nursing journals such as *Nursing Outlook* and *Supervisor Nurse* (now known as *Nursing Management*). The remaining papers were presentations to nursing, healthcare or women's groups. They are presented in their original form, demonstrating her often provocative and fiery speaking style.

The book begins with the paper, "This I Believe about Power in Nursing," which was published in 1973 in *Nursing Outlook* and reprinted in *Nursing Forum*. It was required reading for nursing students and consciousness-raising groups. Describing the "what" and "why" of power, Ashley makes an inspiring call for nurses to individually and collectively cultivate their power.

The second paper, "Power, Freedom, and Professional Practices in Nursing," published in *Supervisor Nurse* in 1975, examines the relationship between medicine and nursing. Ashley argues that nurses, historically subordinated to medicine, have not gained the power and freedom to practice as professionals. She calls for a breakdown in the rigid authority structures in hospitals, the free exchange of ideas in nursing practice, and the fostering of nurse "rebels." The editor of *Supervisor Nurse*, Dorothy Kelly, anticipating a mixed reaction from the readership, urges readers to give the article serious consideration. Her editorial, "The Love-Hate Syndrome," suggests that Ashley's paper presents "a reasoned call for nurses to face squarely their exploitation and misuse and their own more or less resentful compliance with that unethical utilization."

Written for a lay audience in 1975, "Women and the Political Process, Their Social Influence Yesterday, Today, and Tomorrow" addresses politics and its relevance to women. Dr. Ashley discusses the social mythology that has blocked political action by women in the past. She encourages women to use their potential to breakdown barriers and "re-humanize" world society.

One of the most controversial of her papers, "Health Care American Style: Helter Skelter par Excellence," was published in 1975 by *Supervisor Nurse*. Dr. Ashley suggests that evil in our society is exemplified by profiteering in the healthcare system and the continuing oppression of nurses. Far ahead of her time, she calls for healthcare reform. She criticizes the resistance of the medical profession to socialized medicine and argues that the current system of competitive, technology-intensive and disease-oriented care does not match the societal need for healthcare.

Also greeted with controversy, the paper, "Nursing Power: Viable, Vital, Visible," was her keynote address to the 1976 Texas Nurse Association Convention. She again criticizes the state of American healthcare, noting the lack of access for the impoverished and the excesses of medical care, such as unnecessary surgery and overprescription of medication, along with other excesses allowed by insurers. She challenges nurses to break their dependency on medicine and become visible and revitalized in pursuit of revolutionary change. The flood of reaction letters to this paper indicated that Dr. Ashley had indeed stirred the complacency of nurses and generated thoughtful debate.

During the 1970s, nursing gained the right to federal protection for collective bargaining under the Taft Hartley amendments. Nurses exercised their collective bargaining power, showing their political activism. States such as California and Illinois were among the most active in this new political arena. "Nursing Power and Health Care Reforms: The Spirit of '76" was one of the few papers Dr. Ashley wrote in support of unionization efforts. Drawing on the history of oppression in nursing, she suggests that unionization offers the power to liberate nursing. Dr. Ashley urges nurses to examine the structural conditions of nursing work, giving rise to a renewed concern about nursing economics.

The political economy of nursing frames the paper "Professionalism and the Law," presented at the University of Manitoba, Canada, in early 1977. Dr. Ashley extends her analysis of oppression to consider how the law has allowed for the subjugation of power and professionalism in nursing. Drawing on Marxist theory, she relates the contradiction between nurses' education as professionals and employment as laborers to a growing disunity and class struggle in nursing itself. By contrast, the final paper, "Mobilization of Nursing Energies for Constructive Action on National and Local Levels," presents a more conservative analysis and program for change. Written in 1975 for a hospital-sponsored forum for nursing leaders, Dr. Ashley reiterates themes of earlier papers, voicing the need for crisis intervention to end the dominance of medicine and the passivity of nursing. She advocates political action by nurses at the local level beginning with their restitution of control over nursing from medicine. She suggests that nursing explore the development of affirmative action in the hospital setting to aid nurses in upgrading their status and opportunities for advancement.

By the end of the 1970s, political action became an acceptable, if not necessary, component of professionalism in nursing. Dr. Ashley's papers and presentations fueled the momentum to integrate politics into the culture.

Components of Power

by Jo Ann Ashley

The acquisition of power demands a
Loss of innocence.
One pure, one innocent, one free of
Guilt, one free of commitment, cannot
Hope to master the strengths necessary
For assuming the responsibility
    inherent
In the exercise of power.
Loss of innocence is the first, and
Perhaps the most important,
    component of
Real power.
To face the darkness in self and in life
Is to approach the hidden powers at
    your
Command.

Clinging with might to what is deemed
Virtuous and good can only lead to a
Dead end street, a blind alley where
Only the blind gather to chat about the
Terrible weather.
A conscious shedding of one's virtue
Is the path of growing into a mature
Human.
This is the path to power.
This is the path to ethical choice.
Only those who hate can know how to
Love.

Confrontations with good and with evil
Are components of power.
Though knowledge of good and evil
    may
Take you off the beaten track, life
Lived at its fullest must take this
Route.

Knowledge and the beginning of
    wisdom
Involves the passionate consideration
Of evil in self, evil in others.
Only then can the good be freely
    chosen.

Freedom to be is a component of
    power.
Without this freedom, one is doomed
    to
Follow in the footsteps of another.
Beware of where you place your feet if
Your freedom you have not obtained.
You may end up following the very
    devil
And never ever even know it.
Take the freedom inherent in power
    and
March forward making your own way
    toward
Truth and beauty as you seek to create
These in life and in work.

The acquisition of power demands
    knowledge
Of self, knowledge of other humans.
The acquisition of power demands
    knowledge
Of society and the institutions within
    it.
The use of power is the use of self in
Society.
It is the use of self in relation to others.
It is the use of self in coming to know
Self.

Chapter 1

THIS I BELIEVE ABOUT
POWER IN NURSING*

*M*ost, if not all, persons are directly or indirectly interested in power. Some individuals are interested only in their own power and the extent to which it can be used in relationships with other individuals; others are interested in the power overtly or covertly exercised by groups within institutions, communities, and nations. Even the notion of powerlessness implies a consideration of power, for one cannot declare himself powerless without at the same time implying that something or someone else is more powerful.

Professionals, certainly, must take cognizance of the fact that this is an age when increasing attention is being focused on power. Some understanding of nursing power and its use, therefore, is essential in forwarding nursing's interests and goals, in bringing about change, and in responding constructively to change when it occurs.

Many nurses, however, seem to feel powerless or feel that the power they do have is unimportant. Now, more than ever before, a sense of doom seems to pervade the nursing profession. One searches contemporary nursing literature almost in vain, attempting to find articles on the positive aspects of nursing power. Instead, one finds an increasing number of predictions that unless nursing does this or that, it will become obsolete, replaced by something else, or cease to exist.[1-3] And

---

* Reprinted with permission from *Nursing Outlook*, Vol. 21 (Oct. 1973) pp. 637–641.

implicit in all these expressions is a feeling of powerless of inability to control our own destiny.

Such pessimistic utterances can be a demoralizing influence, especially upon students and young members of our profession. When I recently asked a group of senior nursing students what they thought was the most important issue in nursing today, they agreed it was: Will the nursing profession survive? Their rationale for the selection of this issue was "our leaders say nursing may cease to exist." Consequently, their own view of nursing's future was scarcely optimistic or hopeful.

But is "to be or not to be?" really the question facing nursing today?[4] I think not. Instead, since all these foreboding expressions seem to convey a sense of pessimism about nursing's future and powerlessness to do anything about it, we need to start examining power in nursing potential and our conflicts about it. Constantly bemoaning our lack of power is not likely to result in either change or improved professional status. Nor is courage to act constructively at this significant time in our history likely to be enhanced by negative declarations or reiterated fears of nursing's imminent demise. Indeed, a real question facing nursing is: Why do so many nurses express feelings of powerlessness, frustration, and pessimism?

In my opinion, nursing has, and always has had power; it is essentially a social phenomenon and its power derives from society's recognition of nursing as an essential service. The problem lies in the ways in which nurses have used, misused, and abused their power (or failed to use it at all) and in the system in which nursing developed and is now practiced.

THE SYSTEM AND ITS INFLUENCE

Our health care systems, it must be remembered, are the result of years of change growing out of ideas and actions that, in turn, have derived from a basic system of values. It is these ideas, actions, and values that have influenced the development of both medicine and nursing and the social systems in which they function. The desire for power on the part of individuals and groups within these systems has been a factor of no small importance in determining nursing's traditional role and power in the health field.

After all, concerns about power and powerlessness are not new to nursing. Our very history can be described as a power struggle: the struggle to obtain a proper education though opposed by more powerful groups, the struggle to throw off the burden of oppression imposed by those groups, the struggle for the freedom to practice without numerous and professionally extraneous restraints and restrictions. Finally, all of us, at one time or another, have struggled with the need to convince others of the value of nursing and its place in the health care scheme.

Yet how very few nurses over the years have bothered to isolate, confront, and examine the way in which nurses have used their power—not in behalf of nursing, but to maintain the very system that has oppressed them. Instead, current literature dwells upon such topics as "cooperative" teamwork, "collaborative" action, and the interdependence of nursing and medicine. Young nurses quickly learn that they are to use their power, cooperatively and collaboratively, to keep the system operative. They learn less about the ways and means of using their power to change a system that needs changing.

Yet the power to do just that is inherent in nursing. I contend, for nursing power, as a productive force, is the single most important factor maintaining our health care systems today. Without the pooled energies of individual nurses, health care facilities across the nation would be forced to shut down or offer a far different kind of service than they do at present. Unfortunately, however, nurses have permitted themselves to be used as simply a labor force, a means of production, to be controlled and utilized to keep the system and its various parts functioning. Nurses have not been free, nor have they tried to any extent to free themselves, to use their productive powers in the development of nursing.

The association of nursing with production and its free exploitation has had a deleterious effect on the use of nursing power. Although many nurses hold positions of potential leadership and power and engage in constant decision-making processes, few are recognized as appropriate participants in policy decisions. Yet the fact that nurses are the major productive energy in the health field can be used as a powerful force to bring about needed change. Nursing must shed its image of production associated with labor and increasingly cultivate the image of production associated with organized intelligence.

The power of any group is relative, however, and must be understood within the context of the group's proximity to others who have power. There is no question but that many of nursing's conflicts and problems over power derive from the relationships we have established with other groups in the health field. And, certainly, the medical profession is one of the more politically powerful groups in both our society and our health care system. The development of modern nursing has, perhaps, unfortunately, paralleled the development of modern medicine, and the fact alone accounts for many of our difficulties. Medicine obviously has more recognized power than nursing. However, medicine has not always been so powerful, and would not be so powerful, if the medical profession had not managed to control, limit, and use the power of others—notably nursing—to strengthen its own.

MEDICAL AND NURSING POWER

The power that is inherent in nursing was at one time more obvious than it is today. At the turn of the century, the social and professional power of nursing was becoming increasingly visible. Nurses were making hospitals safe for patients, and it was their skills, more than any other factors, that influenced physicians and patients to see these institutions as appropriate places for care. In public health, too, nurses were again a primary force, preventing illness and lowering mortality rates as they applied the principles of their scientific knowledge. The "trained nurses" of that day were highly valued for their expertise, communities as well as physicians increasingly came to feel that they could not do without the most useful professional and humanistically oriented group.

By 1910, the recovery of patients, more often than not, was the result of the nurse's activities and not those of the physician. For example, a surgeon could successfully perform an operation, but without skilled nursing care patients could, and very often did, die of infection. Diet, rest, and "fever sponges" saved more patients with typhoid fever than the medical therapies then available. In lowering mortality rates, nurses were not performing the discarded functions of physicians, they were practicing their own profession and, in so doing, preserving life.

In short, nursing encompassed a great deal more than assisting the physician, and the essential components of the nursing process were carried out without any medical guidance or supervision. Physicians simply were not present to engage in such supervisory activities and, had they been present, they would have had little to contribute to the nursing process. Indeed, professional nursing had not yet become an established part of hospitals and nurses functioned independently in community agencies and in homes.

This is an important point so far as power is concerned, for power relationships involve elements of dependence, and nursing has lived with the myth that it is and has always been the dependent group in relation to medicine. In reality, history shows that physicians very early recognized their own increasing dependency upon nurses. This, and not the reverse, was true.

ALLIES OR DEPENDENTS?

In earlier years, to be sure, physicians had praised the work of nurses openly and referred to them as their colleagues and professional "allies." But this type of colleagueship did not last long because, as nursing power became manifest, physicians came to believe that nurses had to be intellectually and socially controlled. They began to talk about the fact that trained nurses were becoming too powerful and too self-important by organizing their professional association and pretending that they could become a "real" profession like medicine itself.

Historically, such manifestations of power in nursing and reactions to this power led to the development of a peculiar form of communication between doctors and nurses, often referred to today as "the doctor-nurse game."[5] When it first began, however, it was an effort by medicine to control nursing power and minimize nursing's influence. Currently, this peculiar form of communication still serves some function.

Early manifestations of power in nursing also gave rise to present and traditional arguments about whether or not nursing meets the criteria of a profession. The basic issue is really one of power, for those recognized as more expert and more "professional" have more power and more authority. Precisely at the time when nursing organizations were being formed—a significant mark of professional developments—medical men began to argue that nursing was not and could not become a profession. This argument has persisted through the years, and the issue has perhaps consumed more of nursing's energy and time than any other one issue, including ways and means of improving the quality of nursing care and service.

In fact, medical efforts to undermine the confidence of nurses and their power to effect change has been a long-standing source of frustration for nurses. Out of an expression of class interest the medical profession has, up to the present, supported the view that nurses exist to serve physicians and their work in hospitals and elsewhere. The medical profession has also been largely responsible for the content of nursing as a form of supportive labor.

Perhaps even more serious, physicians have encouraged the public to believe that the separate and distinct contributions of nursing really can be attributed to medical skill. Isabel M. Stewart, who was not deceived by medicine's hunger for power over nursing, once spoke of the harm done to nursing, and to its image in the public mind, by the "falsehoods" perpetuated by the medical group. As she explained:

> . . . the same old lies go on circulating years after year, and worse, perhaps, are the hazy half truths which often deceive even ourselves. The difficulty is not, as a rule, that people intend to mislead or misrepresent facts, they are simply unable or unwilling to

think the thing out straight. If we were more familiar with the laws of logical thinking and were determined to tear down every fallacy . . . we should soon get rid of the dead weights of tradition and misstatement which are hampering our progress, and we should have much stronger support from the public in our effort to promote nursing . . . [6]

Nursing has not gotten rid of these dead weights of tradition and misstatement; the public does not generally recognize our need for support. Assumptions, untruths, and myths about nursing abound. Physicians and nurses are not free from the influence of these, either, and both groups help to perpetuate them. The social values of the medical profession have been distorted by their staunch support of a class ideology that has placed no limits or restrictions on their efforts to maintain their power in the health field, very often at the expense of others. And, since nursing has had to work so closely with the medical profession, some of our own values have also become distorted.

Distorted Nursing Values

Many a nurse has used her power to support positions and changes fostered by medicine which could in no way be expected to further the cause of nursing or improve patient care. Indeed, many nurses have unknowingly contributed to the perpetuation of health care delivery systems which have been ineffective in meeting either the medical or nursing needs of large numbers of persons in our society. Nurses, very often, serve as mediators between the system and the consumer; but they use their power to support the former rather than the latter. To the degree that they function as the system's or the physician's advocate, they fail to effect change in the provision of health services to society.

One result of limitations on the use of nursing power has been that the public does not recognize nursing care as separate from medical treatment, needing development of its own to a far greater extent than is generally recognized. More important, many nurses do not seem able to separate the two, either. This lack of distinction and accompanying confusion can be attributed to the beliefs and values underlying the system in which nursing power is exercised. The system itself is based on economic consideration and class ideology. Medical ideology predominates, and class interest and economic gain have been the prime forces impeding change.

For the most part, medical men view themselves as a ruling class. In the past and even currently, doctors are considered authorities on the health needs of people; their ideas are published and they are quoted extensively. The opposite is true of nurses; their contributions and ideas are not made public, probably because so many of them are in production-type jobs and have little time to devote to anything else. In short, nursing power is so hidden and locked in organizations of various types that nursing's visibility is lost to the public and the average citizen has little knowledge of what nurses know or do.

Given this set of circumstances, nursing has literally become the "masses" of, as one physician put it in 1910, the "trained nurse proletariat"—everywhere present, but scarcely an organized force that commands an audience and demands to be heard.[7] Nurses represent a majority in the health field, but a silent one—a majority that is scarcely threatening to the more powerful groups making decisions that can affect nursing's future and the quality and type of care that it provides.

Supporting the "masses" and the labor force concepts is the fact that hospitals and other health care agencies are not unlike large industrial concerns where working class individuals are the largest productive source, and where supervisors, managers, and administrators oversee the performance of these workers in order to ensure maximum and efficient production. Regrettably, there is an analogous situation in nursing, with "supervision" a longstanding characteristic of our profession.

THE SUPERVISION CONCEPT

The concept developed, however, at a time when untrained apprentices rather than fully qualified practitioners were providing most of the nursing care in hospitals. The need for professional supervision of such practitioners has only recently been questioned, and the problems inherent in such supervision are not likely to disappear in the immediate future. Yet I am convinced that the perpetuation of traditional supervisory roles in nursing contributes to the abuse of nursing power. Nursing supervisors and administrators do not always identify with those who make up the ranks of nursing; they more often identify with the powers that be in medicine and hospital management, and this often prevents them from encouraging the development of power and leadership qualities within their own ranks. Such identification is one of the end results of class ideology in the health field.

In fact, class influence and class psychology have had damaging effects throughout the nursing profession. Various groups in nursing often disagree with each other on stated goals and philosophy: they engage in within-group fighting and argue over the merits of their several contributions. Those who make up the ranks of nursing, for instance, do not feel themselves to be the equals of those better educated than themselves or in positions higher than their own in the hierarchy. Feelings of inequality and inadequacy are pervasive.

In short, groups within nursing often act like separate classes competing with each other for status in the system. A collective class consciousness on the part of the total nursing community is largely noticeable by its absence. As a result, collective action on any national scale is almost unheard of, and the powers of the several groups are scattered in many diverse directions. All, however, strive for recognition by individuals in the highest class—medicine.

There is recent evidence that nurses in leadership positions are "least effective" in the areas of interpersonal relations and in communicating with other nurses.[8,9] Interpersonal conflicts abound and serve as an impediment to the exercise of the leadership. Yet if one believes, as I do, that power is inherent in leadership, then it follows that the interpersonal conflicts manifested are really conflicts over the exercise of power. I believe that nurses in leadership positions, more often than not, misuse and abuse their power. Many fail to cultivate a power base among nurses from which to operate. Instead, without communicating with those they represent, they make their decisions in relative isolation and without consensus from those they are supposed to be leading.

LEADERSHIP AND POWER

One result is that the vast majority of nurses have misleadingly been encouraged to believe that they have little or no power. Few recognize the power they do have. Of more serious consequence is the fact that nursing leaders themselves, who have the potential of exercising a great deal of power and influence in our society, dilute nursing power by attempting to operate without a power base. If nursing is to change its image and build up its inherent strength, a different sort of leadership is needed. The power inherent in nursing has probably been most underestimated by the group in nursing. Efforts toward visible demonstration of nursing power will continue to end in frustration so long as nursing leaders fail to recognize, cultivate, and appropriately use their power to effect change.

Paradoxically enough, the medical profession, of all groups in the health field, has not for even a moment underestimated the power of nursing. Physicians have successfully harnessed the power of nurses and used it to advance their own cause, and there is no evidence that the situation will change to any extent in the near future. Today, as in the past, physicians assume that nurses will remain in their "logical place at the physician's side" functioning "under the supervision of physicians" for the purpose of "extend(ing) the hands of the physician."[10]

It is clear, therefore, that nursing's power struggle is far from over. No doubt, physicians will continue to convince many nurses that they are relatively powerless and should not expect public recognition for their professional expertise. If the myth of needed medical "supervision" can be kept alive, nursing contributions will continue to be attributed to medical skill. Those who think that medicine will stop trying to dilute nursing's power and using it for their own benefit are surely naive or misinformed about the nature of power struggles in the health field. Moreover, current efforts supported by nurses to extend and expand the role of nurses may result in further integration of nursing into the practice of medicine, where recognition of nursing's contribution will remain obscured.

Nursing is not and never has been medicine; this fact needs to be better understood by nurses, as well as by physicians and the public. Our powers now and in coming decades should be devoted to changing attitudes—especially the one that sees nursing as simply a vehicle or means of producing that which physicians wish to dispense in the name of health care.

Our national climate seems presently attuned to those who "help themselves." The implications of this seem clear: those who are powerful will be able to help themselves, and those who are weak will suffer. Nursing has been exploited by the more powerful in the past and will be in the future unless we are powerful enough to help ourselves. Nurses, individually and collectively, need to recognize and cultivate the power in an intelligent and organized fashion. The conditions in which we practice our profession in the future depend upon it.

REFERENCES

1. Bennet, L. R. (1970, January). This I believe . . . that nursing may become extinct. *Nursing Outlook*, (18), 28–32.

2. Mauksch, I. G., & David, M. L. (1972, December). Prescription for survival. *American Journal of Nursing*, (72), 2189–2193.

3. Keller, N. S. (1973, April). The nurse's role: Is it expanding or shrinking? *Nursing Outlook*, (21), 236–240.

4. Rogers, M. E. (1972, January). Nursing: To be or not to be? *Nursing Outlook*, (20), 42–46.

5. Bates, B., & Kern, M. S. (1967, October). Doctor-nurse teamwork. What helps? What hinders? *American Journal of Nursing*, (67), 2066–2071.

6. Stewart, I. M. (1921, November). Popular fallacies about nursing education. *Modern Hospital*, (27), 1.

7. Potter, T. (1910, May). The nursing problem. *New York Medical Journal*, (91), 995–999.

8. Hagen, E., & Wolf, L. (1961). *Nursing leadership behavior in general hospitals* (pp. 88–108). New York: Teachers College, Columbia University.

9. Dodge, N. L. F. (1971). *Nursing leadership behavior in the psychiatric unit in the general hospital* (pp. 311–315). New York: Teachers College, Columbia University. (unpublished doctoral dissertation)

10. American Medical Association, Committee on Nursing. (1970, September). Medicine and nursing in the 1970s: A position statement. *Journal of the American Medical Association*, (213), 1881–1883.

Chapter 2

POWER, FREEDOM, AND PROFESSIONAL PRACTICES IN NURSING*

Why build a power base in nursing? In considering the issue of power, this "why to" question is perhaps more important than "how to" questions. Merely seeking power for the sake of having power is not socially a very worthy goal. Nurses hesitant to think in terms of increasing their power may need a clearer understanding of the meaning of power and of its relationship to their own growth and development. Moreover, nurses quite satisfied with their roles and relationships in health care delivery systems may see little need for change. Satisfied with the status quo, some simply do not wish to antagonize either doctors or hospital administrators. They like working with physicians and have not given much thought to how their professional lives have been influenced by hospital administrators.

* Reprinted with permission from *Supervisor Nurse*, Vol. 6, (January 1975), pp. 12–29.

THE WHY OF POWER

In the health field, conflicts over power relationships among nursing, medicine, and hospital administration have constituted a longstanding social problem of major import in providing quality patient care. The basic problem inherent in a lack of power on the part of nursing is that professional practice in the field has remained retarded and underdeveloped. As a result, nurses have not contributed greatly to the scientific knowledge essential for the improvement of patient care. Any group making significant contributions in this area must have freedom and independence to realize their full potential for social development.

Power is most definitely related to both freedom and the self-realization of one's abilities. Thus, to have durable value and meaning any quest for power must be accompanied by serious efforts to relate this search to the need for freedom to enhance productivity on the part of a given group. Without this type of approach to the acquisition of power, nurses may gain it while the true meaning of real freedom escapes them.

NURSING AS A SALABLE COMMODITY

Like health care itself, nursing for most of this century has largely been an economic activity. Providing nursing care has been "big business" and economic considerations have received more attention than the provision of a professional type of care. Nursing has been a valuable commodity, salable in a very nice profit for many institutions. In the selling of nursing service, officials and leaders within institutions have been mostly concerned about saving a dollar or in making a profit; their concern has not been for providing quality care. Commercial nursing homes provide only one example of big business capitalizing on the sale of nursing service. Hospitals are also big business and the primary product they dispense is nursing of whatever caliber they choose to provide.

Within business-oriented organizations the need of individuals to grow in certain directions often takes a backseat to conserving costs.

Thus, providing "efficiency" cheaply while saving a dollar has guided most administrative nursing policy in hospitals. Especially within commercial nursing homes where deplorable conditions of care hurt the reputation of nursing daily all over the country, making a dollar rather than saving one has been the sole aim guiding practice in these agencies. As is commonly known, costs have not been kept down in the health field, nor has the quality improved.

Nursing administrators and supervisors have not been able to escape the economic motivations and considerations involved in the delivery of nursing service. Their charge has been that of staffing institutions as cheaply as possible. Any group of workers (regardless of training and academic preparation) recruited solely to keep a "business" functioning efficiently will soon find themselves losing their incentive to concentrate on the quality of the production they dispense. When costs and economic considerations predominate in influencing staffing patterns, even professionally prepared individuals find themselves functioning like everyone else—putting in a certain number of hours for the monetary rewards provided.

Professional nursing leadership has never had a strong power base in institutions caring for the sick because professional growth and development for nurses has not been congruent with the economic aims and goals of these institutions. Technical (manual) competence and efficiency have been valued. The creative productivity of professionals has not been. The average practitioner in nursing has had neither the power nor the freedom to change this situation. More often than not, even nursing administrators and supervisors are lacking in the power necessary to bring about needed changes. Have the latter really valued change along professional lines? Or have they more frequently been narrowly concerned with planning a budget to please hospital administrators and medical committees? Staffing at the least expensive and deriving both moral and monetary support for nursing innovation and experimentation devalue and exploit the potential of nurses who could constructively improve delivery systems.

Prerequisite to the building of a power base within institutional settings, there must be some understanding on the part of nurses of the extent to which they have been exploited and to which their growth as professionals has been all but stopped. The use of nursing as a labor force has been a major factor preventing the rapid development of professional practice.[1] Viewed as "laborers" (we can say "employees" or "workers" for the squeamish), nurses have not been free to engage in anything but the task of keeping economic institutions operative so that nursing service could be sold around the clock.

As a "jack-of-all trades" who could move from one floor to the next, from one department to another, the nurse has been economically worth a great deal to institutions. Her versatility of technical skill has been more of a monetary asset than her clinical expertise could possibly have been. Recruiting practitioners with expertise will only be engaged in by administrators and supervisors who value the quality of care which can be given only by professional practitioners. Professional practice in any field is primarily an intellectual activity requiring the application of knowledge to the solution of problems. Valuing only technical skills and competency cannot give rise to the growth of intelligent patterns of practice.

POWER AND FREEDOM

It cannot be repeated often enough that the very structure of hospital and institutional staffing in nursing has traditionally been economically and not professionally determined. As a result, nurses have been limited, restricted, and confined to narrow spheres of technical functioning. Too few nurses have questioned the nature of the limitations placed upon them. The vast majority have been, no doubt, contented with their narrow roles. Largely ignorant of their commercial value, nurses have not demanded changes. Contented groups never demand change, they never seek power and freedom in any organized fashion. Any oppressed group happy in a subservient position lacks the incentive to work for change.

Power and its companion, freedom, are never given to oppressed groups. Power and freedom must always be taken. Conformity, blind cooperation and the lack of the questioning of established policies are never avenues to progress or to the attainment of freedom. Nursing leaders have failed both their profession and society by conforming and being cooperative in a system only too responsive to this type of behavior. The average practitioner cannot be blamed for the state in which the nursing profession finds itself. Few in this group have understood that many of their leaders in the fields of practice and education have not valued either professional practice or the improvements in quality which might have resulted from the more rapid development of professionally responsible nurses. Certainly to date, few nursing administrators and educators have valued truly professional practice enough to fight publicly for the conditions in which it could be provided.

It is significant that interest in quality nursing care and specific attention to enlargement of a professional role for nursing within hospitals is little more than a decade old. This trend became evident in the early 1960s and is most clearly associated with the development of clinical specialist roles.[2] Prior to this time professional practice could not be observed within institutions on any wide spread scale. This type of practice could be found in public health where nurses had more freedom to engage in behaviors one could associate with the functioning of professionals.

Power and freedom cannot be considered as separate issues. The struggle for freedom is primarily concerned with resisting the power of any one group to control another. "Control means power," as Perry London has emphasized. Controlling the behavior of a group means, "Power over all the details of people's lives—of attitudes, actions, thoughts, and feelings."[3] To the extent that nurses lack power other groups control their attitudes, their thoughts, and their actions. Since other groups have not valued professional practice in nursing, nurses have not done so either. The best example of this is the one already illustrated in the foregoing paragraphs. Hospital administrators have valued preserving the economy, nursing administrations have also valued this and have permitted groups outside of nursing to influence their actions and decisions in directions unfavorable to nursing's growth.

Moral Considerations

Not only economic considerations have been impediments to the growth of professional practice and freedom in nursing. There are moral, psychological, political, and social factors. Moral problems related to power should be of special interest to nurses. London goes beyond a mere defining of power to discuss the moral and ethical issues involved. As he noted, the real moral problem is that of "how to use power justly."[4]

The meaning of justice and the fair treatment of nurses should be considerations in arguments set forth in support of increasing the profession's power base and freedom. Any brief study of nursing's history reveals a very simple truth—this group has never been treated fairly. Nursing has been exploited, coerced, and forced to develop in directions far removed from a primary focus on professional achievements and contributions. This predicament is not and never has been "morally right." If the members of society understood the treatment traditionally received by nurses, the public would surely come to the support of this group whose freedom to develop has repeatedly been denied them. Nursing can well argue that society could have been much better served if nurses had not been treated in a fashion devoid of any ethical and moral considerations or the meaning of their subservience to more powerful groups.

Traditionally nurses have themselves overwhelmingly viewed it to be "morally right" for them to be self-sacrificing and supportive of other groups in the health field. Their economic exploitation and their subservient role have been universally accepted. Both our health care institutions and the laws of the land have kept nursing in a powerless position. In particular, the legal system has maintained the power of certain groups while serving to keep nursing's power and independence at a minimum. Many nurses have been convinced that it would not be morally right for them to seek rapid change of the legal system or to engage in overt activity designed to improve the conditions in which they work.

The time is now ripe for nurses to re-examine what is morally right and what is morally wrong in the health field. Lack of power and freedom on the part of nurses is a moral problem of major proportions and should be viewed as such. Values are changing in our society. With these changes old habits and traditions should be questioned. Nurses individually and collectively must increasingly arrive at the conclusion that the conviction that it is morally right for them to seek power, freedom and recognition. Members of the profession are responsible to society for what they do or do not contribute through their practice. Yet their right to assume overt responsibility for practice is still not a reality in many settings. Very often, it is the hospital administrator who has the final say on what will or will not be done in nursing practice.

It must be remembered that problems not solved by one generation tend to remain problems decade after decade. It is clearly up to this generation of nurses to claim their freedom and to solve the problems of acquiring the power and recognition already accorded other professional groups in society. Then and only then can professional practice develop as it should. Society will not frown upon our quest for power if we can justify our efforts in moral and ethical terms. The control of nursing's destiny and the development of professional practice depend upon a clear presentation of our motives devoid of the confusion, the misconceptions, and the tears so often accompanying the efforts of groups to obtain their freedom. Nursing administrators, supervisors, and individual practitioners must continuously explain to the public that we do not intend to use power to do harm to patients or to increase the cost of health care. There is ample evidence, if we would use it, to indicate that freeing nurses to practice as professionals improves care and can even cut down on the cost of that care.[5]

PSYCHOLOGICAL FACTORS

Psychological factors are among the strongest impediments to cultivation of a power base in nursing. The greatest of these factors is an outmoded authority. Many authors agree that the climate within hospitals tends to be highly authoritarian. As early as 1948, Esther Lucille Brown commented upon the detrimental effects of the authority structure:

Hospitals predominantly are operated on the authoritarian principle rather than of a cooperative team relationship. The nursing service is caught between the authority exercised by the medical administration, on the one hand, and the hospital administration, on the other. Unfortunately, the nursing service also tends to be highly authoritarian. Hence, the individual nurse finds herself with little freedom or movement and of initiative for other than specified duties, even within the service of which she is a part.[6]

Brown's writings have been quite popular in nursing circles, but her early observation of the problem of authority within the field has received little serious attention. Twenty years after Brown's initial remarks, sociologists were still commenting that nursing was "scarcely autonomous but embedded within a hierarchy of authority" where nurses continue to "look upward to physicians."[7]

That problems with authority still persist is not really surprising when one examines theoretical explanations of the doctor-nurse social system. Supported mostly by the research of sociologists the role of the nurse is described and defined as one in which she would have only indirect authority and power in matters related to the care of the sick. The physician is identified as the "chief authority" while the nurse is viewed as one who assumes an "expressive" or mother role. This role is characterized by the warmth, kindness, willingness to listen and to understand.[8] The importance of the nurse's role lies not in her professional authority or expertise but in her ability to keep the physical environment pleasant while looking out for the common and emotional well-being of all of her patients.

Certainly, a nurse should look out for the emotional needs of patients, but a mother, a sister, a neighbor, a friend, or any good woman can often provide this same kind of care and attention. Seldom is the nurse identified as a person having superior knowledge or expertise similar to that held by other professionals. In the health field, the doctor is viewed as the authority "who must define for the nurse and the patient what must be done in order to get the patient well."[9] Very often the nurse is depicted not as a therapeutic agent but as a mechanical worker who has "lay perspectives."[10]

Sociologists have gotten a lot of "professional mileage" out of doing research on the nursing group. Many of their interpretations are helpful, equally as many are quite harmful to the public image of nursing. Few authors or researchers have utilized psychological interpretations to explain problems existing within the authority structure in the health field (problems which are not solely those of the nurse).

TYPES OF AUTHORITY

Erich Fromm has done extensive work in the area of psychological mental health and the effects of social systems on human functioning. In particular, Fromm has focused his attention on such concepts as power, powerlessness, authority, and freedom in modern society. In regard to authority, he conceptualized two kinds—rational authority and irrational or inhibiting authority.

A study of Fromm's work in combination with my own research has led me to conclude that a system of "irrational authority" has been perpetuated in the health field. It would appear that the exercise of this type of authority is at the root of continuing social problems which impede nursing's progress and which have given rise to public criticisms of the poor quality of health care provided Americans. According to Fromm the source of an "irrational" or "inhibiting" authority

is always power over people. This power can be physical or mental, it can be realistic or only relative in terms of the anxiety and helplessness of the person submitting to this authority. Power on the one side, fear on the other, are always the buttresses on which irrational authority is built. Criticism of the authority is not only not required but forbidden . . . Irrational authority is by its nature based upon inequality, implying difference in value.[11]

Fromm comments upon exploitation and dependency inherent in situations ruled by authorization ethics:

Unless the authority wanted to exploit the subject, it would not need to rule by virtue of awe and emotional submissiveness, it could encourage rational judgment and criticism—thus taking the risk of being found incompetent. But because its own interests are at stake the authority ordains obedience to be the main virtue and disobedience to be the main sin. The unforgivable sin in authoritarian ethics is rebellion, the questioning of the authority's right to establish norms and of its axiom that the norms established by the authority are in the best interest of the subjects. Even if a person sins, his acceptance of punishment and his feelings of guilt restore him to "goodness" because he thus expresses the acceptance of the authority's superiority.[12]

In contrast to inhibiting or irrational authority, Fromm states that:

Rational authority has its source in competence. The person whose authority is respected functions competently in the task with which he is entrusted by those who conferred it upon him. He need not intimidate them nor arouse their admiration by magic qualities as long as and to the extent to which he is competently helping, instead of exploiting his authority is based on rational grounds and does not call for irrational awe. Rational authority not only permits but requires constant scrutiny and criticism of those subjected to it, it is always temporary, its acceptance depending on its performance.[13]

A system of rational authority has not yet emerged in the health field. The expertise (competence or authority) of the professional practitioner in nursing lies in the realm of both the psychosocial and the physical biological aspects of care in health and illness. Yet, how often is the nurse in institutional settings permitted to exercise her full range of knowledge within these domains? The doctor as the identified authority in all areas takes it upon himself to prescribe what will and will not be done for patients.

Physicians have this power and authority despite widespread recognition that medical education has ignored the social sciences.[14] Medical practitioners are not competent in identifying psychosocial needs and problems requiring assessment and solutions. Since nurses are prepared to do this type of assessment, will nurse practitioners emerge as the ones having the competence and authority to do this very thing? It is safe to assume that nurses will not receive wide recognition along these lines unless they can eliminate systems of irrational authority which currently inhibit such professional functioning in practice settings.

BOLSTERING THE SYSTEM

How do nurses themselves perpetuate systems of inhibiting authority? What are some of the psychological factors which prevent change from taking place? Efforts to establish systems or rational authority cannot be as easily observed as self-defeating behavior on the part of nurses. Again, Erich Fromm is most helpful in explaining this phenomenon. Where inhibiting authority operates, feeling of

> resentment or hostility will arise against the explorer, subordination to whom is against one's own interests. But often, as in the case of a slave, his hatred would only lead to conflicts which would subject the slave to suffering without a chance of winning. Therefore, the tendency will usually be to repress the feeling of hatred and sometimes even to replace it by the feeling of blind admiration. This has two functions: (1) to remove the painful and dangerous feeling of hatred, and (2) to soften the feeling of humiliation. If the person who rules over me is so wonderful or perfect, then I should not be ashamed of obeying him. I cannot be his equal because he is so much stronger, wiser, better than I am. As a result, in the inhibiting kind of authority, the element either of hatred or of irrational overestimation and admiration of the authority will tend to increase.[15]

All of the above reactions are prevalent in nursing. There are some nurses who will in private conversation admit their feelings or hostility, resentment and hatred of doctors and or hospital administrators. In the work situation, these nurses tend to suppress their feelings and thoughts because they know only too well that they stand little chance of "winning" anything by revealing what they truly think.

Individuals who express such feelings, however, do not compare in number to those who react by overestimating and admiring the ones who keep them intellectually and professionally oppressed. It is the latter group who have the greater psychological problem. It is this group which will present obstacles to building a power base within nursing. Individuals who repress their feelings because they fear them may actually express feelings of security in dependency roles and will seek to maintain their powerlessness in efforts to remain on favorable terms with those in power over them.

Seeking security in positions of powerlessness and subservience at the expense of freedom, independence and responsibility is not behavior unique to nurses. Such behavior is manifested by all humans and oppressed groups who do not have the inner strength, the will-power or the intelligence necessary for changing their lot in life. Just as slaves in the past feared their freedom, some nurses protest change and fight those who express a belief in the need for it. As mentioned previously, many nurses are quite content with their roles just as they are. To the extent that they are contented or afraid, they will not support any organized effort to increase their power or that of other members of the profession.

The extent to which nursing's position in society is similar to other minority groups is just beginning to be discussed in various kinds of literature. To my knowledge, only one American sociologist makes a specific comparison. Hans O'Mauksch has noted that:

> The nurse, in her interaction with the physician—at least within the work environment—suggests what might be the last vestigial remains of the nineteenth-century relationship between the sexes. In other ways she can fruitfully be compared with the Negro in American society. Reminiscent of the stereotyped views held about Blacks, physicians, when interviewed, will claim that the best characteristics of the nurse are her innate, biologically determined qualities, that she is happiest when working for the physician, and that he, the physician, understands her best and loves her most. This, of course, does not include the "uppity nurses" who, many physicians interestingly believe, are primarily stirred up by outsiders . . . An important aspect of this parallel is that in the work setting, the relationship of the physician is frequently one to the category "nurse"

rather than to an individual co-worker. This perception is similar to inter-caste relationships.[16]

Historical data on the development of nursing and medicine fully support the authenticity of this comparison. Given this type of analysis of the relationship between medicine and nursing, one can further add that those in power may actually both consciously and unconsciously hate the powerless while craving their company because it maintains their feelings of power and superiority over others. Historical documents in medical literature are filled with evidence that many physicians and hospital administration revealed a lack of respect for nurses while at the same time expressing their need for them. To say the least, the relationship among physicians, hospital administrators, and nurses has not always been a healthy one, it has more often been an unhealthy (and unequal) one based on myths, irrational biases, and beliefs. Relationships have been those of master-servant, or superior-inferior. Society has also accepted this view of power groups in the health field. Thus, the problem is broader than the male-female conflicts as observed in practice settings. Nursing needs to build a power base in these settings and elsewhere precisely because of society's discrimination attitudes toward practitioners in the field. If society accepted nurses as professional practitioners (with importance equal to physicians and hospital administrators) and respected their services accordingly, nurses could readily live with the prejudiced attitudes of a local few. However, without power nurses cannot come fully to value themselves and develop the self-confidence necessary for attacking and eliminating societal prejudice directed toward them.

EDUCATION FOR POWER

A main goal of nursing's quest for power must be that of changing society's attitudes toward members of the profession. To do this nurses themselves will require social re-education along with a political sophistication that does not limit its practical application to the support of politicians who hold favorable views toward nursing. The ability skillfully to relate to internal politics in local health care settings, where nursing is practiced needs to be an essential part of every nurse's educational preparation.

Knowledge related to the modes and methods of effective political activism needs to be made available to nurses. This could be a fruitful area for the attention of those in continuing education programs. Those in most need of this type of information are nursing administrators, educators and others who assume leadership positions. Certainly this group needs special consideration if they are to avoid stifling the growth of young professionals who have plenty of knowledge, expertise, and the desire to change the system or health care delivery and nursing's role within it.

Political, social and professional power are associated with freedom of speech and spontaneous action. Freedom of speech for nurses in practice settings is always curtailed and very often derived because of the rigid systems of authority which exist in both medicine and nursing. Creating a climate for the free and spontaneous expression of nursing ideas needs increasingly to become a goal of nursing administrators if they succeed in building a power base. Both formal and informal meetings between staff nurses and supervisors could serve several purposes.

- Exchange of information could remove blocks in communication and help dissolve feelings of animosity between these groups.
- Provide needed encouragement for both as they seek to improve patient care.
- Serve to break down rigid systems of authority which impede the provision of professional nursing in practice settings.
- Provide real evidence that the ideas and viewpoints of all nurses are valued. This evidence alone should tend to decrease feelings of powerlessness.

A systematic approach to the collection, evaluation, and exchange of information and ideas could lead to more creative and more productive means of delivering nursing care. This type of activity might prove to be far more meaningful to nurses than the development of "new roles" for them. "Old" roles within hospitals and elsewhere need to be made more viable and stimulating. If this can be done staff turnover might be lessened to a considerable degree. It is a burden for a profession constantly to be developing new roles for members when the potential in old ones has hardly been realized.

Extending and expanding the role of the nurse may not necessarily result in basic changes in public attitudes. Such roles as they are explained in the literature and are performed in actual practice are only slight modifications of the roles nurses have had in the past. Trying to bring about change by devoting efforts to expansion without devoting equal attention to political and social efforts to gain public support and recognition of expertise already developed is to take the slow route to progress. Nursing can gradually expand its role (as it has always done) and survive another 100 years without ever achieving any marked increase in the power and freedom of its members.

It may be that little significant change is likely until nurses come to view themselves as the equals of other health professionals. So long as nurses admire physicians and hospital administrators excessively and put others above themselves they will always remain subordinate in both fantasy and in reality. External changes in tasks and functions will not necessarily elevate one's self-concept. "To the extent that an individual agrees that he is subordinate and barred from the highest ambitions of the society in which he lives, he will project this attitude into roles he plays and build it into the internal structure of his own psychology."[17]

Medicine, nursing and hospital administration have changed in the past, each has slowly but surely modified its practice. However, at no time in history have nurses loudly and publicly declared that they are the equals of these other groups and that the social values of their professional contributions is of paramount importance. Psychologically, nurses have felt so inferior that they have scarcely been able to make objective evaluations of their own practice and its worth to society. Actually, if one examines the role of nursing in health care delivery systems from a historical point of view, a very good case can be made in support of the argument that nursing's social worth has been the equal of medicine's. Certainly hospitals as institutions could not have survived without nursing service. Now, at a time when society is calling for more attention to the psychosocial aspects of illness, for a more professional, humanistic, and less technical or sterile approach to problems of health and disease, nursing may well emerge as a recognized equal of medicine.

THE NEED FOR ROLES

Is there any one thing that nursing can do to speed up change in regard to our image and our practice? Yes, there is. We need to foster the creation of "rebels" in our midst—rebels who have insightful knowledge, vision, and a cause, rebels with the inner courage to fight for it openly. We need nurses who will fearlessly and repeatedly raise questions about their "place" in established institutions and in society. As Rolly May noted, the "rebel does not seek power as an end."[18] Her (or his) activities are motivated by values, beliefs, and hopes of establishing a better society.

> The rebel insists that his identity be respected, he fights to preserve his intellectual and spiritual integrity against the suppressive demands of his society. He must arrange himself against the group which represents to him conformism, adjustment, and the death of his own originality and voice. Continuously through human history and through the life-span of each of us, there goes on this dialectical process between individual and society, person and group, man and community. When either pole of the dialectic is neglected, impoverishment of the personality sets in. Every man has from time to time impulses to shock his society, fantasies of outraging his neighbors. Paradoxically enough, his own continued mental vitality depends upon this. Also, paradoxically, the community itself, even though it condemns the outrage, gets its health, vitality and new growth from the outrage.[19]

For nursing's health, growth, and vitality we must capitalize on emerging social forces which will aid us in gaining our professional freedom now. Failing to find solutions to moral, economic, legal and psychological problems affecting us can only serve to impede our progress at a time when the societal climate is ripe for a change. Hopefully, from this generation of nurses some independent thinkers will emerge who can intelligently attack the faults in a social system that has lost it social usefulness. The emergence of thinkers who can correct societal misconceptions about us and our goals in society may be the only hope we have of eliminating problems that continuously eat away at nursing's self-esteem. If such individuals do not emerge, future generations will be fighting the same battles that nurses have been fighting for decades.

Society does not yet value independence of mind for women and most especially for nurses. Authority is still the main value subscribed to and upheld in health care delivery systems. It is this very authority that prevents nurses from moving more rapidly toward the goal of intellectual freedom and independence in their practice. If we do not obtain the power to reach this goal, we cannot hope to improve the quality of nursing care made available to the American public.

REFERENCES

1. Ashley, J. A. (1973, October). "This I believe . . . about power in nursing." *Nursing Outlook*, 638.

2. *See* The Clinical Nurse Specialist. New York: *The American Journal of Nursing Company*, 1970.

3. London, P. (1971). *Behavior control* (p. 250). New York: Harper & Row.

4. *Ibid*, p. 251.

5. Brown, E. L. (1970). *Nursing reconsidered: A study of change* (Part 1). Philadelphia: J. B. Lippincott.

6. Brown, E. L. (1948). *Nursing for the future* (pp. 46–47). New York: Russell Sage Foundation.

7. Strauss, A. (1966). The structure and ideology of American nursing: An interpretation. In F. Davis (Ed.), *The nursing profession* (p. 62). New York: John Wiley & Sons.

8. Johnson, M. M., & Martin, H. W. (1966). Nursing: The client and the practitioner. In H. M. Vollmer, & D. L. Mills (Eds.), *Professionalism* (pp. 206–211). Englewood Cliffs, NJ: Prentice-Hall.

9. *Ibid*, p. 208.

10. Freidson, E. (1970). *Professional dominance: The social structure of medical care* (p. 26). New York: Atherton Press.

11. Fromm, E. (1947). *Man for himself* (pp. 9–10). New York: Holt, Rinehart and Winston.

12. *Ibid*, p. 12.

13. *Ibid*, p. 9.

14. Wertz, R. W. (Ed.). (1973). *Readings on ethical and social issues on biomedicine* (pp. 1–12). Englewood Cliffs, NJ: Prentice-Hall.

15. Fromm, E. (1955). *The sane society* (p. 91). Greenwich, CN: Fawcett Publications.

16. Mauksch, H. O. (1972). Nursing: Churning for a change? In H. E. Freeman, S. Levine, & L. G. Reeder (Eds.), *Handbook of medical sociology,* 2nd ed., (p. 223). Englewood Cliffs, NJ: Prentice Hall.

17. Janeway, E. (1971). *Man's world, women's place: A study of social mythology* (p. 108). New York: William Morrow.

18. May, R. (1972). *Power and innocence* (p. 221.). New York: W.W. Norton.

19. *Ibid*, pp. 225–226.

Chapter 3

WOMEN AND THE POLITICAL PROCESS

Their Social Influence Yesterday, Today, and Tomorrow

QUESTIONS ON POWER, POLITICS, WOMEN, AND THEIR SOCIAL IMPORTANCE

What does powerlessness on the part of women mean for them as persons? What would or could it mean for them and for society, if women had the kind of power equal to what we observe men having in our society? If women could rise to power positions as easily as some men do, what would they do with their power? If women truly had political power which was both publicly recognized and accepted on a widespread scale, would they, any more than men do, seek to create a better world? Would their public and private activities serve to re-humanize people and our social institutions more rapidly than we now see occurring?

I have not, of course, answered any of these questions for myself, and indeed, there may be no ultimate answers to them. However, they do require reflective examination by all of us. Thus, I want to share

---

Speech presented to Zonta International, Aurora Area Zonta Club, Aurora, Illinois, April 17, 1975.

53

some of my thinking with you in the hopes that we can have some meaningful dialogue about these and other questions on the meaning of power and politics for women in today's world and in the future.

I will direct my comments to the following areas of concern: (A) the meaning of the politics of living; (B) the political freedom and growth of women; (C) social mythology and our power to effect positive change; and (D) creating a better world, a challenge for women.

The Politics of Living

Politics like a lot of other words has several definitions. It is defined as the "art or science of influencing governmental policy"; also, as "political actions, practices, or policies" (Webster). These are perfectly fine definitions of politics, but to provide a broader perspective I would like for us to focus our thoughts on politics defined as "the total complex of relations between men in society." Now this is a definition taken directly from one of our oldest and most reputable dictionaries used by budding scholars all over the world. This definition does not, of course, mention women nor does it imply that politics includes relations between men and women or between human beings. If the definition had said relations among Mankind (with a capital M), we could possibly conjecture that it meant women too.

For purposes of our discussion and despite its defects, I selected this definition of politics for two main reasons: The first, and obvious one, is that it excludes women and this is the main theme of my paper. And secondly, this definition notes a very basic reality that the political process is a very pervasive and comprehensive one encompassing the total complex of relations between human beings in a society. Politics is a social matter extending well beyond questions of partisan policies and practices condoned by governmental agencies. In human affairs, political processes touch almost every aspect of an individual's life and for this reason it is foolish to ignore or deny the pervasive influence of the politics of living. Since politics implies power, one's political astuteness determines both one's social and one's personal power in a given society or situation.

I would like for us to consider the politics of living as opposed to conceptualizing the political process in a more narrow sense. In recent years, literature from numerous fields attests to the importance of the concept of the politics of living. To illustrate this point, Kate Millet's book on *Sexual Politics* received heated reactions because it was an examination of sexual behavior as portrayed in literature, utilizing a political stance or interpretation. Moreover, much of the current feminist literature refers to the political repression of women, and we can see why this is so since women are even left out of the definition of politics by those who compile Webster's Dictionary with its extensive circulation.

But to go beyond feminist literature, we can see that others are also concerned about the basic question of the ramifications of politics. In psychiatry, for example, Thomas Sasz is noted for his general writings on the implications of politics for the mentally ill in our society. R. D. Laing, another in this field, has written even more specifically on the *Politics of the Family* and *The Politics of Experience*. Within this decade alone, numerous books and articles have been published on the politics of health care and the problems in that field as a whole. Minority groups of all sorts have become increasingly interested in politics.

The literature on the politics of this and that makes for fascinating reading, because those who are not well-informed about political processes are still participants in this process and usually become political victims of oppression by one power or another because of their lack of informedness. It is really somewhat frightening to think that if you are not politically astute about the operations of your own family, you can be driven mad by them; and then again, for political reasons alone, be labeled mentally ill and be put away for life by a society that overlooks the politics of your most human situation.

I wish to emphasize here that politics should be of human concern to all of us since politics on any level involves human behavior and influences on human lives, our own as well as others. When political control rests in the hands of the ignorant, the short-sighted, the ruthless and the powerful whose human interest level is low, lives can be devastated or, at the least, have their true growth stifled. Not only individuals and families, but a whole nation or a society can be victimized by the wrong kind of politics in the hands of inhuman leadership.

POLITICAL FREEDOM AND GROWTH

If women are to avoid situations in which their growth is repeatedly stifled and their lives made difficult, they must become increasingly aware of politics and their social implications broadly speaking, not narrowly in the sense of who shall they vote for in local elections (although the latter is important also). For women, any approach to the philosophical notion or the real acquisition of the good life must begin with an awareness of the full meaning of politics and the accompanying power necessary to live, grow, and realize the highest ambitions they can potentially realize as individuals in a free society. The good life with its full human potential for intellectual and social growth has not been a reality for women in this country, or internationally, precisely because of their naivete about and powerlessness to change political and social orders oppressive to them as a class.

Throughout the world, women have simply not been free to grow as men have in male-dominated societies. For those women who have grown to a realization of many of their potentials, the process of growth has been a struggle, and for some, a burden quite heavy to bear. It is commonly known that professional women in numerous occupations have had to work twice as hard as men to achieve the same status or level of recognition and pay readily accorded men with less education and less experience. The vast majority of women for multiple reasons have not been willing to assume (or could not) the added burden and responsibility for their own growth as persons. A few of us have become professionals, some have remained in the home, while the many have taken on menial and unrewarding jobs out of necessity.

Historically, the failure of women to improve their lot in life has been that of a failure to actively participate in the full political life of the society as a whole. At the turn of the century, women did not have any political status, not even the right to vote. They were not free to actively and openly participate in public debates on their welfare and on the conditions affecting their lives and their work. The early feminists who took on the task of fighting for their political rights were opposed by men and by women as well. These early fighters among our sex were determined, and persisted in their efforts to obtain the right to vote.

They were less persistent in other matters, however. Obtaining the right to vote was only a beginning step in the direction of achieving women's political freedom. A contemporary critic of the early feminist movement has classified the women of the day into two groups, the radical and the conservative. The radical feminists were the most outspoken and the ones who went to jail and endured "embarrassment, mobbing, beatings, even hunger strikes" in order to get the vote. Those radicals who fought the hardest were the ones who were the most politically astute for they also realized that the struggle for freedom could not end with just getting the vote. Their feminist views were characterized by a concern for the total growth of women as human beings, participating equally, with men in the social and economic life of the society with the freedom to realize their highest ambitions.[1]

In commenting upon the behavior of the women classified as conservative in their outlook, this same critic argues that this group was basically non-feminist or anti-feminist in their views. The basic beliefs and attitudes of this group did not seriously reflect concern about the social and political problems faced by women in the society of their day or their rights to fully develop humans with potential equal to that of men. As a result of the influence and activity of the radical group, women did obtain the vote; but as a result of the actions of the conservative groups, they obtained little else with the vote. Upon getting this right, the majority of women went about their daily work and forgot all about the fight for women's real political freedom in all phases of their lives. Thus, women ended up devoting their attention to numerous good causes having little or nothing to do with the elevation of the status of women or to their achievement of equal rights.[2] Women did, in fact, provide visible and invisible support systems for a political and social order that denied them many rights and privileges readily accorded men.

I am most intrigued by this particular interpretation of the outcomes of the early feminist movement for it is in agreement with the findings of my own historical research. Because of the failures of early leaders of both radical and conservative inclinations, we are still fighting for equal rights. And this, as we all know, is a most current political issue. When one generation fails to accomplish what needs to be done, the task is left to be done by future generations. Had our predecessors viewed the politics of living more broadly than they did, we might possibly have equal rights by now. In other words, our work of today was cut out for us by those who lived yesterday. As the common saying goes, hindsight is always easier to come by than foresight and vision, but the main lesson to be learned from a study of history is that of not repeating the errors of the past.

For those of us living now, future critics will examine our behavior and can determine to what extent we influenced our own lives and improved the quality of life for all people, for when human conditions become better for one sex they tend to become better for the other, at the same time or eventually at least. If you buy at all that women failed in the past to better their professional, social, economic, and political status, it behooves us all to look more carefully at how we define the meaning of political freedom for women. If we do not reflect on our definitions and accompanying behavior in this realm, we will repeat the errors of the past and will surely fail again to achieve what future generations might consider desirable. Although we cannot know how they will define failure, we can at least put forth our most intelligent efforts to achieve true freedom while creating a better world in the process.

In regard to historical developments, it is highly significant that professional women, for the most part, fit into the group of those with a conservative outlook. It was the professionals who joined all of the good causes of the day in an effort to develop the social institutions we

observe all around us. In most instances, and with individual excep-
tions, they assumed very narrow positions in taking political action
and devoted their attention, not to changing the social order itself, but
to limited problems related to their own professional development and
to that of their field of interest in local settings. Because of this, women
have not to date made much progress in the professions or elsewhere.

Traditional political positions of professional women require further
study and analysis. Currently, we do know from research exploring the
world of women's work that in comparison to the progress made by men,
"women are falling behind." Significant findings indicate that women
have not been catching up at all over the past generation, but have instead lost ground." Even though, for example, women are more highly
educated than ever before, men are still more highly educated than they
are. Moreover, "women have not displaced or even seriously challenged
male dominance" either in the professions or in the society.[3] As in the
past, the vast majority of women are still relatively powerless today and
politically dependent upon the decisions of men. This, we must admit,
is a reality operative very often both at home and at work (whether the
women are married, divorced, or single).

One of the main points I wish to present for your consideration is that
political freedom is basically intellectual freedom, the freedom to do
one's own thinking. Intellectual freedom and the political and personal
power to make a choice among alternatives go hand in hand, thus the importance of information in a free society. So long as problems and issues
are presented in a one-sided fashion where information is distorted by
dominant persons or groups, or where information is withheld from individuals they cannot know their real alternatives or test the results of
their own thinking, decisions, and actions.

Freedom on any level of living implies accompanying responsibilities for one's choice of action or even of non-action. Exercising one's
freedom to act entails both psychological and social responsibilities.
And who of us, may I ask, with any sense of an independent spirit in
us wants to be responsible for someone else's decisions if we have not
actively and knowingly participated in the formulation of these? Those
who negate the necessity of doing their own thinking do often end up

accepting the responsibility for the errors growing out of decisions not of their making—women are notable for this.

I might add here that freedom does not mean the absence of controls. In particular, "political freedom does not mean freedom from controls. It means self-control."[4] Of necessity, controls are always present in a society, but the nature of repressive societal controls is in need of question by all of us. Those who philosophize on the nature of political thought and action have noted that "whether it be in the field of individual or of social activity . . . [human beings] are not recognizable as . . . [human] unless, in any given situation, they are using their minds to give direction to their behavior."[5]

Most of us would probably be literally amazed if we knew just how little some people use their own minds to evaluate their behavior in a systematic fashion. Traditionally, women, children, slaves, and some free men have all been in the position of being dependent upon others for doing their thinking; in such states, individuals are kept powerless and often used to meet the ends of other people's desires. Inevitably, those in a dependent position, relying upon the evaluations and conclusions of another person's mind, are not and cannot be free or in control of themselves.

SOCIAL MYTHOLOGY AND OUR POWER TO EFFECT POSITIVE CHANGE

Actually, at this point in time, people (both men and women) have less freedom and more outside controls placed on their thinking and behavior than at any previous point in history. In this century, science and technology have become extremely sophisticated and complex. Political processes and intellectual freedom have been greatly influenced by these developments. Partly because of science and technology and partly because of our affluent society (at least for most of us it is affluent), mass conformity is perhaps more of a societal problem than it has ever been. The political reactions of many minority or powerless groups in society are merely a reflection of the extent to which people are getting tired of conforming to faceless machines and faceless people. Powerless groups all over the world are wanting more say over political decisions that affect their lives and well-being.

Many contend that mass conformity is one of the most difficult dilemmas facing all humans. We conform to work roles and to group roles, in both action and thought. Boredom, loneliness, and the fear of acting independently are common to both men and women. Psychological autonomy is a rare finding in persons and social autonomy is almost impossible to achieve, if not completely so. Women and minority groups have taken the route of political action to offset some of their feelings of powerlessness and their lack of control over their lives. Some social analysts have concluded that liberation for individuals and groups will only come through attention being given to the individual's growth with psychological transformation and self-awareness as goals.[6]

Political involvement is surely a must for all. And I firmly agree also that the psychological transformation of individuals is essential this day and age. However, to give perspective on the problems of boredom, conformity, and fears of acting independently, these are not new or merely contemporary problems for women. For this group, they are not an outgrowth of science and technology entirely or to the same degree that they are for men. Such problems on the part of women are more a product of historical oppression and an outgrowth of social mythology. Maintenance of the status quo in the social order, in regard to the roles and position of women in society, has not necessarily been altered by scientific developments. Despite changes, women have continued to assume the traditional roles of wives and mothers or as supporters of men in the work situation. Science has only served to reinforce social myths about women to date, and technology has only added to their boredom because it has provided them with more leisure time in which to be bored.

The boredom and conformity of the housewife and mother have been much talked about since Betty Friedman's unveiling of the *Feminine Mystique.* A more recent book, with which you are probably familiar, provides a far better analysis of the social mythology restricting women's growth than does Friedman's. This book is Elizabeth Janeway's *Man's World, Women's Place*. This author clearly exposes the myths that have bound women to their repressive roles, keeping them from full participation in the life of the society, specifically in the political and economic spheres of activity.

Social myths about women which are old and extremely outdated in meaning and usefulness have not been destroyed by developments in either the social, psychological, or political sciences. A valuable contribution to literature, Janeway's book provides both reason and perspective on why women have not had more power and have not been politically active. Women and the whole of society have been blinded by myths preventing their intellectual and social development as individuals and as a class. Our freedom to grow as beings expected to realize our full human potential has just not been a reality and still is not.

The importance of social mythology and its influence on women, power, and political processes cannot be overemphasized as we seek answers to some of the questions I raised earlier. As Janeway notes, myths are "to be taken very seriously indeed, because they shape the way we look at the world." Moreover, "the urge to make, spread and believe in myths is as powerful today as it ever was. [And] If we are going to understand the society we live in, we shall have to understand the way mythic forces arise, grow and operate."[7] It is our myths that give meaning to our lives.

CREATING A BETTER WORLD, A CHALLENGE FOR WOMEN

As an outgrowth of current feminist activity, we have begun an era of questioning some of the myths so binding to our growth. As we destroy some or all of these, we can expect more favorable changes in women's progress toward freedom and the achievement of their full humanity. As old myths are destroyed, new myths will arise to give meaning to the changes that do occur. This gets me back to my initial point that meaning is what I am most interested in as it relates to this whole topic. Meaning is a myth in and of itself. Just as old myths need to be destroyed, new meaning must arise. What this meaning will be for women who seek power and more political involvement, I cannot say. It will surely be an individual matter in the final analysis.

However, I believe that speculation on the social implications of engaging actively in political processes can aid all of us in our search for new meanings as old ones pass away. The challenge for all of us is that of creating a new world in which the social order reflects more concern for human growth. The main characteristics of the world we now live in are dehumanization and depersonalization. Naturally, boredom, conformity, and fear of independent action are all accompanying ailments. If we can re-humanize this world through political and social action, we can hope to re-discover our lost humanity. Political action and the attainment of power in and of themselves will not serve to re-humanize people or give meaning to life, this we know from experience. Psychological and social transformations are also necessary.

The problems of health, education, understanding, and peace, are human problems requiring the elimination of Mankind's inhumanity to women and men alike. A commitment to re-humanizing world society is a commitment to freedom for all. And "freedom is not an ideal located outside of . . . [the human being]; nor is it an idea which becomes myth. It is rather the indispensable condition for the quest for human completion."[8] Freedom to grow and to be human is not a myth that will become oppressive; real freedom allows for change in myths that give meaning to life. Achieving and helping others to freely achieve a fuller humanity is a service of love of which there is none higher.

REFERENCES

1. Firestone, S. (1971). *The dialectic of sex: The case for feminist revolution* (pp. 15–21). New York: Bantam Books.
2. *Ibid.*
3. Epstein, C. F., & Goode, W. J. (Eds.). (1971). *The other half: Roads to women's equality* (p. 76). Englewood Cliffs, NJ: Prentice-Hall.
4. Meiklejohn, A. (1965). *Political freedom: The constitutional powers of the people* (p. 13). New York: Oxford University Press (Galaxy Series).

5. *Ibid.*

6. Von Franz, M. L. (1964). The process of individuation. In C. G. Jung (Ed.), *Man and his symbols* (p. 245). New York: Dell.

7. Janeway, E. (1970). *Man's world, woman's place: A study in social mythology* (p. 27). New York: William Morrow.

8. Freire, P. (1972). *Pedagogy of the oppressed* (p. 31). New York: Herder and Herder.

Chapter 4

HEALTH CARE, AMERICAN STYLE

Helter Skelter, Par Excellence*

A s we finish the Bicentennial year, we are living in an age of greater and lesser evils. Evils abound all over America in the health field as well as elsewhere. There is enough evil loose in this country to sink the biggest battleship ever made by the hands of man. Many, many persons center their lives around the pure love of evil. In search of pure and simple evil, the major concern of these individuals is that of hoping and praying daily that they will not get caught and publicly exposed for engaging in evil practices of one sort or another. Their primary concern is certainly not that of evaluating the effects their behavior has on the lives of human beings besides themselves. Because of the prevalent existence of massive social evil, we nurses can no longer avoid having serious discussions about this topic which has major influences on our society, our work, our lives.

THE AGE OF EVIL

Prominent and insightful social analysts agree that our age will in all likelihood go down in history as the age of evil. One critic has noted:

---

* Reprinted with permission from *Supervisor Nurse*, Vol. 8, (February 1975), pp. 46–57.

The old ethic of the Judaeo-Christian epoch has proved itself incapable of mastering the destructive forces in man.

. . . the fact remains that man's present state of possession by evil is a phenomenon that transcends political and military frontiers and enters into the hearts of each of us, whatsoever our position may be. The murdered are also guilty—not only the murderer.

Those who saw and failed to act, those who looked away because they did not want to see, those who did not see although they could have seen and those, too, whose eyes were unable to see—each and every one of these is actually in alliance with evil. We are all guilty—all peoples, all religions, all nations, all classes. Humanity itself is guilty.[1]

Since we as human beings may be supporting evil (even murder) without consciously knowing it, we should begin to study evil, preparing ourselves to confront it in self and in others. There is no question of whether or not evil exists. Americans are preoccupied with it. Throughout the decade of the 1960's and during this decade, numerous books have been written on the subject of evil, evil as it appears in our society and in our world today. Some titles (to mention only a few books by social scientists) are: "Sanctions for Evil," "The Structure of Evil," "Escape from Evil."[2] Above and beyond the scientific examination of evil, in our theaters we have movies all about evil. To cite two, "The Omen" and "The Exorcist" have been among the most popular. Today the devil is not only popular, the public is quite fascinated by the whole concept of evil—be it social, public, personal, or private.

EVILS IN HEALTH CARE

We nurses cannot avoid talking about evil for it touches all of us in one manner or another. Throughout this year and all of last, I presented numerous papers on the specific nature of social evils within the American health care system. We have brutality and violence everywhere in the form of unnecessary surgery, drug abuse, and malpractice in general. We can read in the newspapers daily about the misuse of the federal and state monies going into health care. The exploitation of the public by the American health care system continues unabated, with no end in sight.

In addition to corruption and violence, we have the social evil of the severe oppression of nurses. The political, psychological, and social repression of nurses is a favorite pastime of many hospital administrators and physicians; nurses, too, repress other nurses. This particular social evil has been a characteristic feature of the American health care system for over a century. American style health care has in essence meant this: oppress nurses and exploit the public to make a penny or a dollar.

The jackpot of funds in health care has gone to the powerful and the greedy. The latter are the businessmen (including physicians and hospital administrators) who have operated and controlled health care facilities mostly for commercial gain and for private profit. Because of the American way of oppressing us nurses, very little money has filtered down into our hands for use in improving nursing practice. Our existence within the system has been one of surviving from decade to decade, from day to day, with little real support and planning involved where our welfare is concerned.

The economic game played in the American health care system for over a hundred years has never been a fair game. In a fair game all participants have at least a chance to win. In the health field, the game is more or less fixed. The winners are winners from the start. These winners are the powerful who have much, but continue to gain, precisely because they have power and the financial means of keeping it. In contrast to other groups, we nurses have had to crawl like worms to make every inch of progress we have made over the years. Nothing has come easy for us—not our education and not the improvements we have managed to make in both practice and education. In modern times, this maltreatment of the nursing profession constitutes a social evil of unbelievable and disgraceful proportions.

Because of the major role played by nurses in health care, nurses deserve an equal share of the goods and produce derived from the delivery of services, especially nursing services. The profits in health care have gone to a select few for too long now. We should, as individuals, and as a group, be very tired of a competitive game in which the rules are blatantly unfair, unfair to us and unfair to the public.

Since we have been oppressed to the extent we have, nurses have shaped nothing in the health care system. In reality, we have not shaped anything in nursing either. Instead, we have been shaped by laws, ideas, politics, policies, and practices not emanating from us nurses. The paternalism we have lived with (and that we do live with now) has not allowed nurses freely to shape a thing. As a result, we have very little to be proud of within our profession or within the American health care system. As we all know, we have had problems controlling and influencing our social destiny. As nursing literature so clearly points out, we have, for some time now, had problems with our "identity" as professionals. Out of fear and frustration, some nurses even express the view that nursing will not survive. The inability of nurses to shape our own development has had profound effects on all of us and on the public as well. Nursing care is the heart and the core of health care; and so long as nursing is manipulated, exploited, abused, and misused, we will not see quality in care improved in this country.

Historically, we nurses have lived with a dog-eat-dog competitiveness characterized by a lack of real and meaningful planning on both national and local levels. Moreover, the economic philosophy of individualism and accompanying laissez faire approaches to delivering medical care have had pervasive effects on hospitals, on nursing, on medicine, and, of course, on the health of our society. Always fearfully opposing favorable changes, the medical profession in particular has sought to avoid what they have called the "evils" of socialized medicine.

To this day, some among the public, along with professionals, fear what is labeled "socialized medicine"; and yet, there is no clear definition of what socialized medicine would turn out to be in this country. Socialized medicine cannot be equated with federal spending in health care because we have had this type of spending for some time now. I might add here, no one at all has been opposed to socialized nursing, which should give us nurses food for thought as to why this has not been an issue in the past.

Irrational fear, such as that surrounding the concept of socialized medicine, gives rise to social evils not clearly examined by anyone. This has been the case in health care. Fear and the greedy disposition of dominant groups in the health field have given rise to a state of delivering care in a helter-skelter fashion. The term "helter-skelter" means to function haphazardly; it means to function in haste, in "hurry and in confusion;" it means to move forward or backwards in "headlong disorder" and in "turmoil," without pause or reflection. So says the dictionary. American style medical care, nursing care, and health care have all been delivered in a hit-and-miss fashion.

Solving problems in this manner has dehumanization and waste as the major outcomes. In other words, historically and currently, crisis intervention has been the favorite method of trying to bring about change in health care. This type of intervention has not resulted in favorable improvements in the past and it will not work in the future. It has only led to the creation of one crisis after another.

As nurses, we all know crisis intervention as a method of treatment merely takes care of emergency situations and surface conflicts; it does not have long-range curative effects because it does not really involve getting to the roots of what is causing a crisis. To further illustrate this point, I will give you an example of what I mean by crisis intervention or helter-skelter efforts to solve crippling problems in the health field. A few years back, the proposal was made that the introduction of new health workers would solve the health care "crisis." Workers such as physicians assistants and other allied health workers are now prominent groups in the field.

Common sense alone tells us that the addition of new workers with varying levels (and sometimes unknown levels) of educational preparation will only make more confusing and more complex the problems with which we have to deal. Adding new categories of workers has led to increased economic competition for scarce monies. This development has led to numerous social evils in the realm of greater fragmentation of care, with increasing depersonalization and dehumanization of patients at the hands of the incompetent. This has also intensified the ever-existing problem of social discrimination directed toward nurses. The introduction of new workers was accomplished in a hurry and in confusion. It was a form of short-sighted crisis intervention destined to create new problems, not solve old ones.

Many tend to think that national health insurance will solve current and future crises confronting us. However, as nurses we must remind ourselves that numerous fraudulent practices surround the pouring of unregulated federal monies into health care. Physicians, drug companies, commercial nursing homes, and hospitals have all had quite a glorious time exploiting both patients and the government. As proposed now, national health insurance will eliminate none of the social evils we can observe in health care.

Of primary importance to all of us nurses, the various proposals for correcting defects in American health care grossly devalue the worth of both nursing care and nurses. Moreover, none of the proposals being implemented, or those on the way to being implemented in the future, is even remotely innovative. None will accomplish the changes needed in order to get at the root causes of distress and poor health within our society. Instead of blindly accepting the short-sighted thinking so prevalent today, we nurses must become more critical and outspoken on issues so vital to us and to the public.

SOCIAL PATHOLOGY IN SOCIETY

In our American health care system, we have the situation of greater evils joining hands with lesser evils—a state in which social evils are dominant. In this situation, science and technology have won and human beings have lost, a loss having very damaging effects on the health of our society.

All of you have surely heard of John Dewey. He was a very fine philosopher who made many astute observations about our society in the early stages of its massive industrialization. He made one predictive or future-oriented observation which has come true in health care. He commented in 1916:

When the acquiring of information and of technical intellectual skill do not influence the formation of a social disposition, ordinary vital experience fails to gain in meaning while schooling . . . creates only "sharps" in learning—that is, egoistic specialists.[3]

This is precisely what has happened in health care. We have too many egotistical specialists of all kinds in medicine—technical-minded, machine-like individuals who cannot see or hear the human beings they treat. Following in the footsteps of medical men, we have egotistical managers who know nothing about health or nursing care; the latter only know how to identify with the powers that be in medicine, and their concern is most often power and money, not care, not humans. It is this type of individual who is the real "devil" in the American health care system.

I cannot emphasize strongly enough that more disease-oriented medical science, more technology, more managerial rigidity by those with no "social disposition" will never solve our problems in health care. To support more of any of these is to support social evils that can only lead to more social evils of a greater nature. It will be to support the greatest evil outcome of all in the form of devaluing the importance of nursing care.

Like John Dewey, we nurses need to begin making astute observations about what is wrong with our society. We need to set our sights on correcting some, if not all, of these wrongs. We need to begin shaping ourselves and our destiny. We need to begin the slow and tedious process of creating a different kind of society, a society fit for humans to live in freely with a minimum of psychological, social, and physical distress. We cannot eliminate all distress, but we should at least prevent that distress which can easily be prevented by professional nursing care.

Here, I wish to provide an example of some of the wrongs we need to consider. I recently had the experience of being pressured into thinking about societal evils, evils I did not want to think about at all. My graduate students kept asking me to read a book entitled

Helter-Skelter. My students were insistent. They wanted to know if I thought the book had any implications for nursing and for health care in this country. You are probably familiar with this book. It is a book all about evil. It is a book all about poor, unhealthy people. It is a book all about children: children unloved, children abused, children unwanted, children hated by their parents and by society too.

Written by a lawyer (Vincent Bugliosi), this book is, in my opinion, inappropriately named. If this book had been written from a nursing point of view, the nurse author would not have chosen the same title as the lawyer did. A nurse would surely have entitled the book something like the following: *Children of Death in a Modern Age,* or the *Outcomes of Social Pathology in Children Needing Nursing Care.* The lawyer's title also seemed inappropriate since most of us Americans live our lives in a helter-skelter fashion. As I have said, our entire American health care system is conducted in a helter-skelter fashion. The murders described in the book *Helter-Skelter* were not done in a helter-skelter fashion; they were well-planned.

This book about evil, about children and their sometimes unfortunate fate in the world really deals with health and nursing problems unseen by society. Both the murdered and the murderers had health problems; the lawyer as author made this quite clear. One of those murdered was in need of prenatal care at the time of her death, and one of the murderers even had the urge to preserve the life of the unborn child, or at least had feelings for the unborn infant. The killed and the killers could have profited from human nourishment before and at the time of death.

The social and personal sicknesses depicted in this terrible book could have been prevented years ago if we lived in a society that valued nursing care and made it available to those who are desperately in need of it. All of the wicked parties depicted could have been made into healthy and useful members of society if they had received intelligent nursing care when infants and thereafter as needed.

Unmet nursing needs were really the causative factors giving rise to the pathology so blatantly revealed by the planned murders of individuals in California, so recently recorded as current history. A society producing this type of pathology and violence, especially in children, is not a healthy society. Like my graduate students, the fact that children can so easily be destroyed, and taught to destroy human life, bothers me. It bothers my students and me because we are professional nurses. As nurses we know that pathology of the kind described can, in most cases, be prevented with proper nursing care and attention.

The reading of this book about evil forced me to raise a number of questions: *In what way is society to blame for such evil? In what way are the courts and the prisons to blame? In what way are the psychologists and the law officers involved to blame? In what way can the American health care system be blamed? Must the nursing profession share guilt when problems in needy children go undetected—problems in children who are young, homeless, and without a mother who is fairly decent and healthy?*

As nurses, we must raise questions like these and attempt to come up with answers that satisfy our urge to know what is human and what is not human in our society. These types of questions are very much related to the place of nursing care in society. Nursing is human nourishment and when it is lacking in the lives of persons who need it this lack gives rise to evils, great or small. We must confront the issue of how much nursing care is respected and sought after in our society. To what extent is nursing care paid for by our societal institutions when nursing care is clearly indicated as the means of more healthy life styles for self and others? Without high quality nursing care, the old, the middle-aged, and the young are destined to suffer unnecessarily, with needless and painful death often the outcome. Without high quality nursing care, societies and even civilizations cannot survive and be truly healthy.

THE EVIL OUTCOMES OF OPPRESSION

More disease-oriented science and technology are not the means by which we can correct defects in health care and eliminate or make less the social evils we see manifested in persons and in institutions. We must go a step further than just spending money on science and technology. Right now within America's health care system, technology in the hands of men without social and ethical dispositions is being utilized to kill not to cure. As you must know by now, unnecessary surgery has been publicly exposed as a serious health problem, posing fiendish difficulties for all of us in nursing. This is no minor problem for society either. If we think the murders reported in the book *Helter-Skelter* were bad, we need to look more closely at what goes on in the health field. With medicine recognized as a potential killer in surgery and in the abuse of drugs, we nurses have serious thoughts to think.

As professional nurses, we are all quite familiar with operating rooms. Many of us spend long days and long nights in them. We have always thought of these rooms as rooms serving the useful purpose of providing space for saving the lives of the sick and the wounded. We can no longer solely think this way since, in many instances, these rooms have become death traps for some of our youngest and our most healthy citizens. The murders committed by children in California were planned; they were not done in a helter-skelter fashion like the statistical deaths reported for healthy persons seeking help from money-hungry and technology-oriented specialists in the medical field.

It is we nurses who have to care both for the victims and for the legitimate surgical patients who come out of operating rooms in hospitals across this country. The rather sordid and messy situation in the health care system will increase the workload of nurses for some time to come. Patients, and potential patients, will experience more and more anxiety when confronted with hospitalization, especially surgery, however minor; and we will have to help them deal effectively with their feelings of fear and well-grounded apprehension. This will take extra time and extra nursing energies.

Even more important than the time element, nurses should be incensed at the very thought of being unknowingly forced to cooperate in the provision of care that is not care at all. As professional persons, we must ask ourselves how guilty we are as accomplices and as supportive figures participating in certain ugly acts taking place in the health care system. We must engage in a more searching examination of the root causes of dehumanization as it appears all around us in the places where we work. We ourselves have been dehumanized to a point where our very own humanity is at stake. Most of the nurses I meet and hear from by mail feel frustrated, hopeless, helpless, and oppressed. We are not, at the moment, in very good shape. Too many nurses have ceased to feel alive. They have ceased to feel or to act as humans.

In thinking of our oppression, and the effect this has had on the lives of nurses, I cannot help but recall the words of Edwin Markham who wrote of the ugliness of oppressed humanity. This writer urges us all to ask: "whose breath blew out the light within this brain . . . who made . . . (the oppressed of the earth) dead to rapture and despair, a thing that grieves not and that never hopes."[4] Although we nurses have been severely oppressed, we still can, and do, feel despair. For some, however, the light has been blown out of their brains, leaving only darkness and no more.

As nurses, we have had to contend with a social evil forcing us to live within a culture of poverty. According to Maxine Greene and other contemporary authors, a major problem in our society is the very real phenomenon of "the culture of poverty." As Greene noted, this is "a concept first used by anthropologist Oscar Lewis in his efforts to understand poverty as a way of life which is passed down from generation to generation along family lines."[5] To quote her further:

> This culture (or, more technically, subculture) takes form among certain poor people who happen to live in a success-oriented capitalist society. These people do not and perhaps cannot achieve the upward mobility valued in that society and are therefore considered personally inferior or inadequate because of their lack of success.[6]

As an oppressed group in work life, nursing fits very aptly into the category of those coping with a "culture of poverty," assuming the role of beggars and living in constant fear of not surviving. To date, we have not been fully recognized as a group having much to offer society, separate and apart from our association with medicine. As a result, society has not supported us and we have, in many respects, remained poor. As a professional group, we have been crippled and handicapped by poverty in spirit and in purse.

It is time for us nurses to take a totally new look at the social evils shaping us into what we have become. We need to get a clear perception of our place in society today. In order to use our energies effectively in the future, we will have to shed all of our illusions and put ourselves in the category and class where we have already been placed by society, by the medical profession, and by managers in health care facilities. Our culture of poverty must be examined by each and every one of us, both female and male nurse.

As a silent majority in the health field and in society, we can remain silent no longer, not at home and not at work. Climbing out of poverty and oppression will not be easy; it will mean that each nurse as an individual must begin to shape herself (or himself) into a responsible human quite capable of changing self, society, and our profession's social destiny.

As we engage in meaningful dialogue about the social evils confronting us, we may need to throw away our textbooks, our procedure manuals, and our rigid ways of thinking and acting. Many, many nurses are fearful and afraid of emotions, afraid of interpersonal confrontations. It is time to shed our fears and assume flexible attitudes toward self and toward other nurses. As we begin to grow away from oppression, we will need to demonstrate a bit of kindness, a bit of compassion, and a bit of patience toward one another. For the truth of the matter is that nurses do not necessarily like or respect other nurses. This attitude is not unique to nurses; it is a common feature of all oppressed groups.

THE USE OF ART IN OVERCOMING EVIL

Having confrontations with evil should be the goal of all of us nurses now, and in the near future. To gain perspective on directions for new kinds of growth toward humanness, we need to look at evil in ourselves and in others. Perhaps the worst evil we nurses engage in is that of being afraid of our emotions, being afraid to act forcefully. Our greatest evil is surely that of conforming to a system of health care that dehumanizes both us and the public. Conformity and the fear of emotions and feelings go hand in hand, stifling the very life within humanity.

Oppression instills fear; it makes people less than human. In the movie, *One Flew Over the Cuckoo's Nest,* the nurse is portrayed as a non-human being having a face of stone and a heart of steel. She appeared to have no feelings, no emotions. Many of you have surely seen this movie and recall the scene where, because of her inhumane responses, the nurse is being choked by a patient. During this particular scene, in the theater where I saw this movie, people in front of me were calling out "bitch," "bitch," and behind where I sat, people literally screamed, "kill her," "kill her." Hearing and seeing this reaction, I grew quite cold inside. There I sat as a nurse hoping no one around would, or could, know I was a nurse kin to the one they wanted killed at that moment.

I left the theater that day and went home to think some serious thoughts. The movie had not amused me. The emotional reaction of ordinary citizens to the nurse with the heart of steel got through to me. I had, and could understand, some of the same feelings they had expressed, but at the same time I understood the nurse, too. I knew there was a real-life story hidden behind that movie. The portrayal of that awful nurse was most realistic. I know nurses like her who go to work in psychiatric hospitals every morning, evening, and night. Moreover, I know our educational programs have, in the past, taught nurses to behave in the manner depicted by the actress—to be cold and objective is professional, so we have been told. Such education has not been a good, but an evil. It is oppressive and can only lead to hard-heartedness in the one who receives it. Individuals so trained cannot have, and do not have, any compassion for humans in distress. They do not have a social disposition of the kind John Dewey was talking about.

In the assertiveness training movement of today, women are being urged to avoid the "compassion trap."[7] However, we in nursing cannot avoid this trap because compassion and feelings for our fellow human beings are the core of nursing practice. By compassion, I do not mean the act of playing some stupid, silly, pleasing game motivated by dependence needs and weakness, both associated with outdated womanly qualities. In our oppression, we nurses have been forced to assume this role in the past. We should refuse this role in the future. As we truly move away from being shaped by others and begin to shape ourselves into the humans we can potentially be, we can learn how to show compassion intelligently, out of a sense of strength and power.

In this age of evil, we live in a society that worships science and technology. We need to grow into a society that more fully appreciates the art of being human. As nursing practitioners, we should spend a good deal of time reminding ourselves that people are not machines, and we nurses are not machines either. It is time a number of nurses at all levels of practice become more concerned about the artistic side of nursing practice. I say this because it will be the nurse as artist who will develop concepts most relevant to the subject of what it means to be human, a kind of knowledge sorely needed in nursing and in our society today.

In the health field, we need to turn away from an exclusive praise of science and dwell more on the meaning of art. Susanne K. Langer defines art as "the creation of forms symbolic of human feeling."[8] Art, and art alone, teaches one not to suppress, repress, or kill the feeling side of life—the side of life that is most human. More than ever before, society needs the nurse as artist, whether the nurse applies knowledge from the arts or engages in artistic creation. Valuing human feelings and human worth is an absolute necessity in our field, and this is precisely what is lacking in health care. American style.

In recent years, societal values have changed and one of our main problems is that we ourselves, and we as a profession, have not caught up with the changes which we are being forced to deal with. This matter of dealing with changed values, and most of all the prevalence of evil, is not one of choice; it is one of necessity. To further elaborate upon this point, the Russian author, Alexander Solzhenitsyn, has raised questions about dealing with changes in values:

> Who will coordinate these scales of values, and how? Who will give mankind one single system for reading its instruments, both for wrongdoing and for doing good, for the intolerable and the tolerable, as they are distinguished from each other today? Who will

make clear for mankind what is really oppressive and unbearable and what, for being so near, rubs us raw—and thus direct our anger against what is in fact terrible and not merely near at hand? Who is capable of extending such an understanding across the boundaries of his own personal experience? Who has the skill to make a narrow, obstinate human being aware of others' far-off grief and joy, to make him understand dimensions and delusions he himself has never lived through? Propaganda, coercion, and scientific proofs are all powerless. But happily, in our world there is a way. It is art, and it is literature.[9]

Not only Solzhenitsyn but a number of individuals and writers are suggesting that we as a potential world society need to return to a more humanistic view of mankind, of humanity. We need to do this in our local hospitals and in all of our health care settings. Where nurses are concerned, our compassion must begin at home with ourselves and our beaten profession; it must begin where we live and where we work.

The cultivation of a new and emerging humanistic viewpoint will entail a re-examination of the term art as it relates to nursing practice and to health care. An intensified interest in the arts is a societal development having major implications for us nurses. As another author has pointed out, this movement back to the arts

. . . indicates that modern . . . (humans are) now reaffirming . . . (their) own existence in the dehumanized environment which . . . technology has created. It is not sufficient, however, for us merely to proclaim that we do indeed exist. It is necessary that we be capable of giving substance to our life; and we can do that by learning to make contact with the dimension of depth that is at the core of our being.[10]

As professional nurses, we need to reaffirm ourselves as human beings worthy of living, and living well, in this society. We need to stop expressing our constant fears that we will not survive and get busy making sure that both we and the art of nursing will survive and be financially supported far more than we or nursing have been in the past. Both our art and our science depend upon our gaining more affluence, and more leisure time, to spend in cultivating the knowledge and feeling base of our practice. After all, society can scarcely do without our profession and the human nourishment it provides to the sick and the well.

We nurses have been losers for too long now and society has suffered as much as we have because of it. Nursing is the very backbone of the American health care system and we are the only group who can preserve what is worth preserving in the system as it stands now. Though our own back has been bent by oppression and economic exploitation, it is time we stood up and walked tall to a winner's position.

As we begin to pause, to think, and to reflect more seriously upon just who we are, we will change our tune in nursing. Instead of yelling and screaming disunity, or deploring our lack of identity, we can sing a different song altogether. Pretty soon the public will hear us and will surely respond to us differently. It is time societal values reflected a desire to preserve the lives of those humans who happen to want to become more useful as contributing members, functioning in opposition to destructive elements having no good end in sight for any concerned citizen.

Confronting the evils I have discussed in this paper is a must for us nurses. The only way for us to confront evil is to hang onto intelligent compassion and to our own human dignity. Then, we can set out to openly fight those evils that prevent humans from receiving the human nourishment that only nurses can give as a full-time professional activity.

Considering the most obvious health problems within society now, we need to be saying, along with the popular singer, Dory Previn,

> give me your poor
> your maladjusted
> your sick and your beat
> your sad
> and your busted
> give me your has-beens
> give me your twisted
> your loners
> your losers
> give me your black-listed.[11]

We cannot, however, sing this type of song until we move away from being oppressed losers ourselves. We nurses have been black-listed for a century, and for the sake of the people who need us, we must rid society of this evil.

REFERENCES

1. Neumann, E. (1973). *Depth psychology and a new ethic* (p. 26). New York: Harper & Row.
2. *See* N. Sanford, & C. Comstock (Eds.). *Sanctions for evil*, San Francisco: Jossey-Bass, 1973; E. Becker. *The Structure of Evil*, New York: The Free Press, 1968; E. Becker. *Escape From Evil*, New York: The Free Press, 1975.
3. Dewey, J. (1916). *Democracy and education* (p. 10.). New York: Macmillan.
4. Markham, E. (1958). The man with the hoe. In R. J. Cook (rev. ed.), *One hundred and one famous poems* (p. 55). Chicago: The Reilley & Lee Co.
5. Greene, M. (1973). *Teacher as stranger* (p. 183). Belmont, CA: Wadsworth.
6. *Ibid.*
7. Phelps, S., & Austin, N. (1975). *The assertive woman* (pp. 34–43). Fredericksburg, VA: Bookcrafters.
8. Langer, S. K. (1953). *Feeling and form: A theory of art* (p. 40). New York: Charles Scribner's Sons.
9. Solzhenitsyn, A. (1972). *Nobel lecture.* Translated from the Russian by F.D. Reeve. (p. 17). The Nobel Foundation.
10. Progoff, I. (1963). *The symbolic and the real* (p. xv). New York: McGraw-Hill.
11. Previn, D. (1972). *On my way to where* (p. 92). New York: Bantam Books.

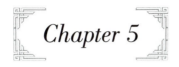

Chapter 5

NURSING POWER

*Viable, Vital, Visible**

*I*n this Bicentennial year, America is not beautiful. In particular, within the American health care system, our red, white, and blue flag blows in the breeze over a very ugly sight. Because of defects in health care, the fathers and mothers, and the sons and daughters of America are not as healthy or as happy as they could be. Our society is not a happy one; it is not a healthy one.

Let me elaborate on the ugly sights causing our society to be less than a happy one and less than a healthy one. I will outline for you some of the damaging effects growing out of our sick medical care system. By now it is commonly known that numerous abuses derive from the practices of incompetent medical doctors. Large numbers of the public are oversedated, over-medicated, overdrugged by careless physicians who do not wish to spend time dealing with the real problems manifested by patients seeking their help.

* Reprinted with permission from *Texas Nursing*, (August 1976), pp. 11–18.
Editor's Note: This is the text of the keynote speech Ms. Ashley delivered at the 1976 TNA Convention. It is controversial. It has to make intelligent readers think. Reader response is welcomed, in fact, expected. The best will appear in a future issue of TN. In introducing her keynote speech, Ms. Ashley said, "I believe in freedom of thought, speech, being. . . . You don't have to believe what I say. If you don't, throw it in the trash basket of your mind. Your time is too precious to waste it on what you don't believe."

Drug Abuse

As the newspapers tell us, thousands of people are killed each year by faulty drug prescriptions. Most recent evidence indicated that "Every year . . . 30,000 Americans accept the drugs their doctors prescribe for them and die as a direct result." Studies reveal "perhaps 10 times as many patients suffer life-threatening and sometimes permanent side-effects, such as kidney failure, mental depression, internal bleeding and lost of hearing and vision."[1]

According to *The New York Times* "these figures are among the more conservative." But the figures are immense as they are, conservative or not. The realities of gross defects in health care are there and we can no longer deny them. As the *Times* points out, even "most medical authorities agree that some of these deaths and near-deaths could have been prevented if the doctors involved had exercised better judgment in prescribing drugs for their patients."[2]

The prescription of unneeded antibiotics and tranquilizers by ignorant and uncaring physicians is only one area of abuse. Unnecessary surgery and accompanying death is presently a national health hazard of major proportions. The findings of the Congressional subcommittee revealed that "at least 11,900 surgery-related deaths occur(ring) in the United States last year were entirely avoidable because the surgery involved was not necessary."[3] Other sources of data comment on the costly nature of the death of healthy Americans, since unnecessary operations are now costing the public "close to $5 million a year and kill(s) as many as 16,000 Americans" a year.[4]

As we all know from recent publicity, within the nursing home business the elderly are oversedated and subjected to various kinds of cruelty. The book *Tender Loving Creed* published in 1974, provides more than ample data on the extent to which the provision of real nursing care is being derived to citizens.[5] While well-educated and highly qualified nurses remain unemployed or while some move from one job to another year after year, the aged go without care because of the employment policies and practices of nursing home owners.

The abuse in these agencies has been labeled an American "scandal." And here it is a scandal because the elderly are victimized and their money taken while no nursing care if given in return. At best, many, many nursing homes are staffed by housekeepers, untrained aides, or LPNs. Here in this situation, we have large numbers of the population totally dependent upon the unmerciful care of the ignorant and the incompetent, and is often supposedly supervised by an equally ignorant and incompetent physician who knows little or nothing about the nursing care of the elderly.

The highly publicized abuse of the public by uncaring physicians is all the more appalling since, as nurses, we know that hundreds of people and even thousands of them go without needed nursing attention in this country of ours. Unexplored health problems lie hidden and buried in the homes of families and in the minds of individuals who could lead happier and more productive lives if professional nurses were available and paid to help them with their difficulties and with their concerns.

A Case in Point

To illustrate this point, I am now involved in the teaching situation where the clients we see are poverty victims, having the unfortunate experience of being dependent upon "public aid." Most of these victims are women with large numbers of children, children fathered by numerous men who may not reside in the household. These mothers and their children live in a county in Illinois that has no public health department and no county nurse. There are no public clinics either.

The system of delivering medical care there is the familiar one of private enterprise controlled by local physicians. And there is, of course, no nursing care provided at all. The county will not recruit and pay a professional nurse to provide nursing care to members of the community who cannot afford a private physician. The system there is worse than archaic, it is inhumane.

Even small babies in that county (and in several surrounding counties) are deprived of being immunized because physicians will not permit or will not support publicly sponsored programs of immunizing children. The physicians argue that such programs are not needed. They also argue that citizens do not want this type of care. Their real reasons for opposing these programs are, of course, economic ones. A mother has to be wealthy enough to have her own private physician before she can get her children cared for decently. Even with a physician the care she gets can hardly be considered decent or adequate with nursing care still a missing part of that care. As you can guess, many, many mothers and children receive no care at all.

With the condition existing in any part of this country where indigent women and children are deprived of both nursing and medical attention, we can scarcely conclude that we live in a healthy society. The truth of the matter is that in that section of Illinois, which is rural farm country not far from the windy city of Chicago, the cows, the sheep, and pigs are better cared for than are many human beings. The cattle in that part of the country are beautiful and obviously healthy. The farmers may well be wealthy (at least some of them are) and I am sure they immunize their cattle as often as this service is needed.

Reality Is Not Pretty

In your imagination, travel with me to another state, the state of Kentucky. I recently went to Kentucky to visit my parents who live in a small place near Mammoth Cave National Park which is, as you know, beautiful country. However, conditions in health are not so beautiful there right now. To my surprise, I learned that the two "country" doctor services in my native home country are engaging in the same practices as the "city" doctors. This practice is the abuse of drugs. I was told by neighbors and friends of my parents that nearly everyone going to those doctors are given tranquilizers of one sort or another, young and old people alike. These are honest people like you and like me, who earn their living by working. They do not deserve the poor quality of health care they are getting.

Upon leaving Kentucky, I drove back to my place of work in Illinois somewhat sad and somewhat angry. In reflecting upon the beauty of Kentucky's blue grass and its race horses, I hated the ugly sights I saw in health care there. I hated the poor treatment being received by good people. In thinking further about our lack of progress in health care of the years, my memory went back to the time when I was a student nurse doing my tour of duty in public health on the outskirts of Louisville, one of the largest cities in Kentucky. During that public health experience, I saw children with potbellies playing on dirt floors while dying of starvation.

The wise and experienced public health nurse who accompanied me as a teaching supervisor told me that when she first started her practice in public health nursing her heart was broken by what she saw about her. She also said that for the first few months of her work in public health she spent her paycheck to buy food for starving youngsters. She did this until her husband finally told her to stop it or quit work. He told her she was crazy to behave in such a manner, wasting her hard-earned money. Her husband was right, of course, since this single nurse alone could not hope to feed the starving children of Kentucky. She could not by herself alone make a dent in the societal problems of poverty and starvation. She was powerless. Her hands were tied, preventing her from fully practicing the art of science of nursing, a kind of care sorely needed by those she served.

Nurses Have Role

I have shared these observations with you for one main reason: There are many scandals associated with health care delivery in this country of ours. As nurses we must begin to publicly expose more and more of these scandals and gain public support in getting some, if not all of them, corrected. The scandals and the poor quality of care being provided the public cannot be corrected until the vitality and visibility of nursing care is more fully appreciated and supported by the American public. We have scandals in health care because we live in a society where nursing care, separate and apart from medical care, is grossly devalued.

As we all know, our systems of paying for health care very often negate the need to pay adequately for nursing attention by qualified practitioners. With the devaluation of nursing a major societal problem, it is time we nurses listened more closely to outspoken critics of our American health care system, critics who claim that physicians have ceased to be "healers" and have become the creators and sources of many new kinds of disease. I make specific reference here to work of Ivan Illich who has just recently embarked upon a study of what ails health care systems in this country and elsewhere. Illich makes the charge that professional medicine has become a "major threat to health."[6] Certainly, in view of the problems I have cited, medicine has become public menace number one, in many respects, it has become a destructive force in our society.

At this time, the public identification of medicine as a threat to health should be of special interest to us nurses. It should be of interest to us because historically medicine has served as a destructive force attempting to prevent the delivery of decent nursing care to the American people. I am, as a professional nurse, making the assumption that nursing care of the highest caliber possible is absolutely essential and vital to any kind of quality in health care. As nurses we know this to be true. Since this is so, we can surely agree that any group or societal force powerful enough to prevent the delivery of quality nursing care presents a threat to health and is a destructive force.

THE BIRTH AND SLOW DEATH OF NURSING'S VITALITY

Now that I have examined the decay which can be observed in the American health care system, I will move to a discussion of nursing's vitality and what has happened to it in the past century. I wish to emphasize one point here, the predominant position of medicine and management in health care have obscured the role of nursing. The giant positions of these two groups have stifled both the vitality and visibility of nursing, keeping our vital importance from being fully understood by the public. The truth of the matter is that nursing has always been devalued by medicine and by managers in the health field. This has been continuously true throughout our history. And this is still true. In contrast, medicine itself has been idolized to the point of a disgraceful worshiping technical and chemical cures which have become a monstrous problem, killing off almost more people than are cured by them.

In any consideration of nursing's vitality and the ways of using power to foster our future growth along favorable lines, it is extremely important for us nurses to fully understand the manner in which medicine and hospital managers have repeatedly tried to stifle and oppress nursing over the century. To help explain this process of oppression and the behavior of physicians and managers, let me make a distinction between the terms viability and vitality.

Viability and Vitality

A thing that is viable has the presence of life within it. To be viable is to be alive, it is to give promise to growth and more growth. Viability may, however, imply only a state where growth to full potential never becomes a reality in fact. One of the best examples I can think of to illustrate this is that of the newborn infant, a most viable creature, but one very much dependent upon mother for moving beyond the point of mere survival to vital growth toward real maturity. The infant gives promise of growth, it contains the seeds of growth within body and mind but its state of dependency renders the infant merely viable at birth.

Another example illustrating the difference between the concept of viability is that of a seed that contains the possibility of growing into some kind of tree, a tree capable of producing seeds of its own. The seed when planted is merely viable, continuing only the potential for growth. As with the infant, conditions of the soil, the climate, the care, and attention received are important determinants of just how the seed may, or may not, grow into a well-developed tree.

Self-actualization and the realization of viability leads to a state of vitality. Unlike being merely viable, vitality is the actual experiencing of growth, maturity, and the rewarding productivity associated with this. Vitality implies the conscious exercise of one's strength in making choices about directions to be taken in growth. Vitality implies the use of personal power, and collective power, in achieving growth in self and in others, be they clients or colleagues. Vitality cannot become a reality with limitations and restrictions placed on one's thought and upon one's ability to engage in constructive actions. Vitality cannot become a reality in a climate and in an atmosphere unfavorable to growth.

I am spending time on these distinctions for two main reasons: First, this is the theme of your convention; secondly, when you as individuals leave the convention returning to your various practice settings, get in the habit of continuously asking yourself if you are feeling your viability, your vitality, or are you feeling nothing. If you conclude that you fit into the latter category of feeling nothing, you will know for sure that you are more nearly dead than alive. Should you find yourself in this state, do not get alarmed, just remember that a physician cannot help you at all. You will need nursing care, so talk to yourself or consult with your nurse colleagues. You will begin to feel better almost immediately. Nursing care in the form of human nourishment can do wonders when one's vitality is seeping away and one is nearly dead while still alive.

Society Defined Caring Roles

Having made these distinctions, I will elaborate upon what I call the birth and slow death of nursing's vitality that many of us nurses are trying to make alive, real, and visible in today's world. In the case of us nurses, we have been subjected to a most harmful process of systematic oppression, providing you with a poor historical climate in which to grow. Our most powerful opponents have been medical men, those in private practice, those in organized medicine, and those in management positions in hospital and other health care settings. Medicine's powerful position in health care can be partly explained by use of the family as a model of relationships, with masculine and feminine members. At the birth of modern nursing, the family was the institutional model for the operation of hospitals. As a result, nurses assumed the feminine role and physicians assumed the masculine role with all the privileges accorded men.

Nurses actually assumed "wifely" and "motherly" duties in caring for the hospital family, especially its male members. The age-old myths about women and their relationships to men determined the characteristics and the nature of nursing's relationships with others in the health field. These myths were not, of course, based on a factual examination of what women needed in order to move from a viable beginning profession into one making vital contributions, contributions of equal value to those made by men in their professions. Helping the nursing profession realize its vitality has not been a goal of our society, not in the past, and this is not a priority goal in the present either.

From our earliest beginnings, both in the minds of nurses and within the minds of leaders in our societal structures, nursing has been married or tied to medicine. We have been tied to medicine ever since nursing first came on the American scene. This has been for us a relationship of subservience and of powerlessness stifling to our growth. As women, supporting and protecting men was built into the professional and technical activities of nurses. These protective and supportive activities have been a major part of the work carried out by individual nurses and by the profession as a whole. Our relationship has consumed so much of our energy that we have had little left for developing our own art and science of nursing practice. To date, as a discipline, we are a bit retarded because of this.

Nursing Smothered Itself

The progress made in medical science, and the dominant role assumed by medicine, could not have become realities if this group had not had the vital support and protection of nurses. As women in the home have kept the house in order while men worked and made progress in the professions, nurses have kept house in the hospital so that medicine and hospital managers could do the same in their professions. In other words, we have helped others cultivate their vitality and their power over us while our own power and vitality was being slowly smothered and choked to death right before the very eyes of us nurses. We have all, every one of us, felt this smothering process.

The concept of women as the supporters of men's vital functions in the world of work has very clearly been operative over the century in health care, as in other fields of work. The feminine functions of nurses have actually shaped the development of American nursing. One of our most outstanding nurses, Isabel M. Stewart noted that this concept of nurses and nursing fostered the "tradition that men are naturally superior to women, and that women exist mainly to serve the comforts of men, and that men know best what is good for women, whether in politics or education or domestic life."[7]

The feminine role and functions of nurses have kept us from moving forward in an independent fashion; this lowly role has kept us from moving beyond the state of mere survival to the desired state of real vitality. Nursing has always been most viable because nursing care is absolutely essential to the survival of societies and of civilization. However, tied into an unhealthy relationship with medicine, nursing has been made legally, economically and socially somewhat dependent upon this group when this need not ever have been the case since nurses can function far more independently than can physicians. Had we historically been in the climate more conducive to the freedom and growth of women, we would never have become dependent upon medicine at all.

Medicine: Dependent on Nursing

With nurse playing "wifely" and "motherly" roles, helping medicine grow instead of nursing, medicine has always been far more dependent upon nursing than has been commonly realized by nurses and the public. Physicians themselves recognized this dependency very early. The expression of increasing vitality on the part of the nursing profession at the turn of the century caused physicians to fear that nursing would become an independent profession. As these fears of nurses' independence increased, medicine's desires to control nursing and nurses also increased.

Historical fact demonstrates the extent to which organized medicine refused to communicate with leaders in nursing. Physicians must have thought that ignoring this group and refusing to support developments in nursing would serve to stifle the spirits of nurses who were striving for professional status equal to that of the physician. Organized nursing was ignored. Medicine reacted to nursing as if the profession itself was little more than an object to be used in the service of medicine and in the service of hospitals; hospitals, not as centers for nursing practice, but as the workshop of physicians.

The majority of physicians and managers of hospitals denied the full worth and potential of nurses and engaged in both public and private denial of the fact that professionally qualified nurses were an essential element in the treatment, care, and recovery of patients. And we, as contemporary nurses, are still living with the social consequences of this type of destructive behavior. The ugly sights we now see in health care are an outgrowth of this destructive behavior also.

Cast in the "servant" and in the "domestic helper" role, we have been unable to climb up to a position of equality with medicine, to the detriment of us nurses and to the detriment of the public's health. The words of a physician, W. Gilman Thompson, best illustrates the predominant view medical men have had about the nursing profession for a century. As Thompson stated:

> The whole question is this: Is nursing a subordinate profession to medicine, or is it a separate, distinct, and independent profession, which when it gets old enough and big enough, is going to sever every connection with medicine and set up as an entirely separate science and art?[8]

Nursing was doing so much social good at the turn of the century that medicine began to fear the seeds of potential growth displayed by this infant profession. At the time, there was no question whatsoever about the viability of nursing. The profession gave promise of much growth. It was the right of every nurse to grow from a state of viability then evident to a state of vitality then possible. It was the sight of the nursing profession as a whole to do the same. However, medicine and others in society sought to deny, and did deny, nurses that right.

Myth of the Holy Marriage

The relationship between nursing and medicine has been one based on what I call the myth of the holy marriage between nursing and medicine. Because of this myth, physicians assumed that nursing would always remain tied to medicine as a legal, subservient partner. Because of this myth, we nurses were taught that we belonged "under" medicine. Because of this myth, our societal, political, and legal systems "placed" us "under" medicine.

The myth of the holy marriage between nursing and medicine was held to be sacred and fixed. This myth implied that nursing should remain lower than medicine in the health care hierarchy. Despite the ingrained nature and strength of the myth, physicians still had many fears that nursing would separate itself from medicine, becoming an independent profession. This historical fear (and current fear) on the part of physicians is no different from the concerns of the worried husband who fears that if his wife becomes educated and independent she will leave him for greener pastures. This has been the fear of the century on the part of physicians. When relationships between the sexes are changing, this is a common fear expressed by men. This has been so down through the ages and it is still so.

In the quote illustrating the medical profession's attitude toward nursing, Dr. Thompson did not stop by just stating the question about independence and the fear that nursing would separate itself from medicine. He went further and expressed some of the more typical beliefs held by the average physician and the average hospital administrator:

> A fundamental error obtains in attempting to designate the occupation of a nurse as a profession. It is a profession in no proper sense of the word, which "implies professed attainments in special knowledge, as distinguished from mere skill." The work of a nurse is an honorable calling or vocation and nothing further. It implies the exercise of inquired proficiency in certain more or less mechanical duties, and is not primarily designed to contribute to the sum of human knowledge or the advancement of science.[9]

Though nursing was considered the lower half of medicine, keeping nurses in an inferior and limited position was repeatedly urged in medical literature. The following statement from *The Journal of the American Medical Association* clearly illustrates continuing efforts to dominate and to restrict the actions of nurses:

> Every attempt at initiative on the part of nurses . . . should be reproved by the physician and by the hospital administration. The programs of nursing schools . . . should be limited strictly to the indispensable matters of instruction for those in their position . . . The professional instruction of . . . nurses should be entrusted exclusively to the physicians who only can judge what is necessary for them to know.[10]

Keeping the nurse in her "proper sphere" and in her limited "province" was declared to be the duty of both the physician and the hospital administrator. Physicians repeatedly argued that nurses

> should cultivate a pleasant temper, cheerful countenance and encouraging demeanor . . . She should never attempt to appear learned and of great importance . . . In addition to these fundamental essentials, she should be able and willing to render intelligent obedience to the instructions of the attending physician and carry out his orders to the letter.[11]

Another quote illustrates the intense desire of medical men to rule over women in nursing and control them with an iron hand. As medical men put it:

> The education of the trained nurse for obvious reasons should be under the supervision of the medical profession and hospital nurse superintendents and head nurses especially, the subjects of intelligent official control.[12]

Nursing did survive in this type of atmosphere, but the vitality of nursing and its growth to full potential as an art and a science has not yet become a reality. We have not as a result achieved professional equality with men in medicine. Also, a most damaging outgrowth has been that our visibility is scarcely favorable in the public's mind.

Nurses: A Subordinate Subject

Of notable significance historically, our leaders in the key positions of nursing service directors and head nurses are referred to as "subjects." According to Webster's dictionary, a "subject" is "one that is placed under authority or control" or a subject is "one who lives within the territory of . . . and owes allegiance to a sovereign power or state." Only a slave or a person in a very servile status is likely to be referred to and treated as a "subject" in need of constant and "official" control.

In the minds of physicians, the nursing profession was characterized as being "essentially subordinate" to medicine, a dictum not to be questioned. As one physician put it:

> In the sick room and operating room the general orders, the fundamental, essential, controlling things, are expressions of the needs, wishes and scientific demands of physicians, not of nurses.[13]

The views of medical men and hospital administrators have been most damaging to the welfare of nurses, and damaging to the public's welfare. Also in the twenties, the president of the A.M.A. in a speech at their national convention, emphasized that "the proper work of the trained nurse does not contemplate that she is in a position of primary responsibility . . . The things she has to do are simple things."[14]

The public has been brain-washed by comments such as this. "Subjects," slaves, and domestic servants have traditionally been considered "simple" souls and good-natured objects designed for use by others. In the thirties, this view of nurses is clearly expressed in the words of the president of the American Hospital Association who emphasized that nurses did not need higher education because to educate them was like educating a "people beyond their sphere of usefulness." This particular physician and hospital administrator went further stressing the point that nurses should, he strongly believed, "enter the (nursing) profession for the love of the work and the good they may do."[15] Not unlike a wife or a mother, nurses were to work out of a sense of love, and out of a sense of being professional and economically rewarded for their vital contributions to the well-being of society.

Efforts to stifle and to kill viability and vitality are clearly associated with oppressive systems and with social prejudice, be it sexual or racial, knows no bounds when it comes to putting and keeping people in their places. The French woman, Simone de Beauvoir, who wrote the classical document, *The Second Sex*, noted:

"The eternal feminine corresponds to the black soul" . . . there are deep similarities between the situation of woman and that of the Negro. Both are being emancipated today from a like paternalism, and the former master class wishes to "keep them in their place"—that is, the place chosen for them. In both cases the former masters lavish more or less sincere eulogies, either on the virtues of "the good Negro" with his dormant, childish, merry soul—or on the merits of the woman who is "truly feminine"— that is, frivolous, infantile, irresponsible—the submissive woman. In both cases, the dominant class bases its argument on a state of affairs that it has itself created.[16]

Just as the black slave was supposed to remain merry and happy despite his deplorable position in life, the nurse was supposed to do the same and never complain. As I mentioned earlier, physicians expected nurses to "cultivate a pleasant temper, cheerful countenance and (an) encouraging demeanor" despite the miserable lives many nurses lived in their oppressed state.

THE CONSTRUCTIVE USE OF NURSING POWER

Make no mistake about it—within health care nurses have been the "coolies" and the "donkeys" of the system. In countries where there are well-defined caste systems, a coolie is a "cheap laborer" or an "unskilled" person of very low status. We all, of course, know what a donkey is, but as this relates to us, we nurses have been treated sort of like "domestic asses." Laboring under the myth of the holy marriage between nursing and medicine, this has been our lot in the world of work. Lacking in real vitality, and lacking in any real opportunity, to achieve it, we have, in many instances, been viewed as if we were little more than a beast of burden or a work horse.

In studying the history of nursing's oppression, I have had to remind myself time and time again that "dogs" are men's best friends, not women and not children of either sex. We can read in literature and hear in conversation men talk a lot about "top dogs." I have concluded that all this concern for dogs by men has not helped our society much. Certainly, because of the poor treatment given us nurses and our profession, health care in American society has completely gone to the "dogs." The "top dogs" are the physicians and the managers of care facilities. These groups, because of their social class and their power, have easily maintained the position of "top dog."

Letting medicine and managers remain in dominant positions in health care has resulted in errors (in both policy and practice) having lethal effects in their outcomes. Both nurses and the public might ask: What animal doctor would give a poor dog tranquilizers and antibiotics just to get that poor dog out of his office and off his back? What animal doctor would take out the uterus of a female dog just to earn "rent money?" The latter is, as you may or may not know, a common practice among some specialists where women are concerned.[17]

Social Injustice

The nature of basic problems within the health care system is one of social injustice and misguided values. We are not a classless society and the health care system is only one unhealthy system reflecting the detrimental effects of class boundaries that keep certain groups in positions that prevent them from realizing their vitality where power, visibility, and deserved recognition are concerned. As nurses, we must be serious about wanting power. We must be serious about getting power.

Social injustice in the health care system calls for nothing less than revolutionary changes, changes that cannot be accomplished without a great deal of nursing power.

As nurses, we have been taught to be loyal to the physician. We have been taught never to say an unkind or critical word about him in the presence of a patient. We have been taught never to question his judgment in any way, form, or fashion. For the nurse to do so, it has been argued, might result in the awful possibility of undermining the patient's confidence in his doctor. The psychological effect of such teaching has been that of instilling fear and inhibitions within many nurses. We have remained silent even when we knew Mrs. Jones would most likely die because her doctor happened to be Dr. Jones. The social consequence of such teaching is the present phenomenon of healthy and not so healthy people dying in wholesale fashion from drug abuse and from unnecessary surgery initiated by the hands of uncaring physicians.

Change Is Possible

To revitalize nursing and to obtain the power we need to bring about constructive changes, we nurses can no longer remain loyal to the physician or to managers. Our health care system has been and is a patriarchal system operated on the principles of an authoritarian ethic. It is a system in which liberty and freedom for us nurses have been lacking. We must reject the soundness of the system and replace it with better creations through which to serve the public's health needs.

Two assumptions have influenced the survival of the patriarchal system we know as health care. Assumption number one is the belief that women should, and would, remain psychologically and legally tied to men. Assumption number two is the belief that women exist to be exploited and to remain in the lowest, and in the most powerless, positions possible in society. These are assumptions we must question and no longer accept.

The goal of organized nursing in this Bicentennial year should be that of revolutionary change. The energies of nurses at the state and district levels in our organization should be directed toward bringing this type of change about. Power is energy used effectively to bring about change. Each individual nurse at the local level is a unit of energy. She is a precious unit of power. In viewing individuals as units of energy and as units of power, we can go a step further and think in terms of pooling this energy, or this power. Our professional organization is our source of pooled energies. It is through the use of ourselves and through the use of organized effectiveness that we can increase our power on national, state, and on local levels.

MAKING VITALITY AND VISIBILITY REAL

It is through the process of working for revolutionary changes that we will make the vitality and visibility of nursing real. Let me make the meaning of revolutionary change clear as it applies to nurses and to the health care system in this country. To be specific, I mean this: It would be a revolutionary change if we nurses psychologically separated, or divorced, ourselves from medicine long enough to cease being their supporters, protectors, and accomplices in perpetuating the mess we now have in health care.

It would be a revolutionary change if we nurses were recognized as the equals of physicians and given the support we need to function as professional persons. Realizing this would really only be a matter of social justice, but since we nurses have not had fair treatment in the past achieving this now will be a revolutionary change.

It would be a revolutionary change if we nurses became active as equal participants in the shaping and in the making of health care policies on both national, state, and local levels, serving on hospital boards, on community health boards, and on national committees.

It would be a revolutionary change if our most highly educated nurses were paid differential salaries in all hospitals across this land. It would be a revolutionary change if these same nurses were given the freedom to practice professional nursing and to do research that is adequately supported and financed. It would be a revolutionary change if hospital managers and boards of trustees began to truly value nursing practice enough to employ our best prepared to be directors of nursing service departments and paid them salaries comparable to those paid to the chiefs of medical and surgical services.

These revolutionary changes I have identified are, I repeat, only matters of social justice which we rightfully deserve in this democracy of ours. To date, justice has not been made by mankind anywhere on this earth. To achieve justice we need the active, the public, the conscious input of women in health care, this input will come from the women in nursing, or it will not come at all.

Nursing's Obligation

Vitality breeds viability and this leads to visibility. Visibility is itself a sign of constructive and positive growth. It is the public evidence that one's viability and vitality have not been stifled by lethal forces that would kill life rather than help it grow.

Viable, vital, and visible we want to be. Society needs us in our most healthy state. At this convention and in the coming year, keep saying to yourself (as an individual and as an organization), our time has come to have power to use for the good of our society. As nurses, we want our place in the sun, a sun that casts no rays of discrimination across our path, or across the path of another human being.

It is high time that the dark night of discrimination against, and abuse of, our sex and our profession came to an end. Power must be used wisely if we are to find our place in the morning's sun of growth, realizing our full potential. It is we nurses, and it is our profession, that can make America and its people more beautiful in the coming years. Our obligation to society is that of seeing to it that people get the human nourishment they need to live, to grow healthy, and to grow happy.

At its founding, our country and its people were beautiful. It needs to grow beautiful again. To do this, our country needs nothing more or nothing less than nursing care of the highest caliber possible. Let us get power and use it to give our country this.

References

1. Rensberger, B. (1976, January 28). "Thousands a year killed by faulty prescriptions." *The New York Times*, 17.
2. *Ibid.*
3. Brody, J. E. (1976, January 27). "Incompetent surgery and needless death found not isolated." *The New York Times*, 24.
4. *Washington Post*, Washington, D.C., July 16, 1975.
5. Mendelson, M. A. (1975). *Tender loving greed.* New York: Vintage Books. Originally published by Alfred A. Knopf, Inc., 1974.
6. Illich, I. (1971). *Tools for conviviality* (p. 2). New York: Harper & Row.
7. Stewart, I. M. (1921, November). "Popular fallacies about nursing education." *Modern Hospital, 17*(2).
8. Thompson, W. G. (1906, April). "The overtrained nurse." *New York Medical Journal, 83*(845).
9. *Ibid.*
10. (1906, December 1). "Nurses' schools and illegal practice of medicine." *The Journal of the American Medical Association, 47*(1835).
11. Beates, H. (1909). *The status of nurses: A sociological problem* (p. 6). Philadelphia Physicians' National Board of Regents.

Chapter 6

NURSING POWER AND HEALTHCARE REFORMS

*The Spirit of '76**

* Presented at the Annual Convention of the United Nurses' Associations of California, San Diego, California, October 18, 1975.

THE THEMES OF DOMINATION VERSUS LIBERATION

*O*ne of the most challenging tasks confronting us nurses today is that of gaining both social and historical perspective on our position within the American society and within the health care system. This is an essential first step in initiating action to increase the nursing power necessary for advancing our cause in bringing about needed reforms in nursing and in health care.

Reflecting upon just who we are and upon the history of our profession can serve to give meaningful direction to the efforts we invest in creating a better society in the future, a better society not only for ourselves as nurses but also for the public we serve. Since our history is one of oppression, we need to understand the nature of this oppression more fully in order to overcome certain myths and illusions which bind us to the past and undermine current attempts to improve our situation.

Within our society right now, a number of diverse groups are all clamoring for more power, or shall I say, they are insisting upon their liberation from powerful forces and groups that dominate their lives. Women, blacks, and various ethnic and minority groups are seeking to have their humanity recognized by our society. To give some perspective on nursing's place in this significant social movement, we are a large, diverse group composed of not only whites, blacks, and Jews, but also women from every ethnic group one can name. We now have men entering the profession in increasing numbers as well. We are as diverse as society itself.

I want to emphasize our composition for one main reason: we are an extremely complex group. Our complexity as a social group and our age are factors we must consider in mobilizing our power-base around issues of importance to all of us alike despite our diversified ethnic backgrounds. We all have one thing in common, we are members of the nursing profession and that profession is an oppressed group. Because of our oppression we have all been treated as a minority group. We have had more than our share of problems related to prejudice, to powerlessness, and to a variety of conflicts both of a social and psychological nature.

Because of who we are, one of our major priorities this day and age must become that of understanding and respecting each other as individuals. Our power to liberate ourselves and our profession depends upon this respect and this understanding. Though some may well disagree with me, I do not believe we will truly gain a sense of unity until we are well on our way to liberation from the dominating forces that continuously impede our progress.

As I see it, the move toward liberation and the move toward unification can occur simultaneously. This is to say, one condition does not have to wait upon the presence of the other condition for our forward advancement. Given our complex diversity as a group, if we wait for a perfect state of unity or agreement, we are likely never to achieve our freedom and independence as a profession.

A contemporary author of the book entitled *Pedagogy of the Oppressed* has observed that "the fundamental theme of our epoch . . . [is]

that of domination—which implies its opposite, the theme of liberation, as the objective to be achieved."[1] As this author notes, oppression is dehumanizing. Historically, we nurses have been grossly dehumanized and are still being dehumanized by dominant groups, groups that will not seemingly face the fact that we need to be liberated now and not at some future point in time decades away.

In view of current opposition to reforms in nursing and in health care, the major themes I want us to think about today are domination and liberation. To help explain these themes for us nurses, I am going to provide you with some historical examples of issues that are a century old in nursing. But, before examining specific aspects of our history, I want to clarify what an understanding of our history can do for us. The historian, William Appleman Williams, succinctly states the value of history for those who care to reflect upon it:

> History as a way of learning has one additional value beyond establishing the nature of reality and posing the questions that arise from its complexities and contradictions. It can offer examples of how other . . . [human beings] faced up to the difficulties and opportunities of their eras. Even if the circumstances are noticeably different, it is illuminating, and productive of humility as well, to watch other . . . [humans] make decisions, and to consider the consequences of their values and methods. If the issues are similar, then the experience is more directly valuable. But in either case the procedure can transform history as a way of learning into a way of breaking the chains of the past.[2]

What we nurses need to begin to do is to break a few chains of the past. In order to do this, as Williams emphasized, we need to examine the values, beliefs, behaviors, and decisions of our counterparts of the past who dealt with the same issues that we are dealing with today. In order for us to examine past and current problems in nursing, I will comment upon the following two issues: The first is that of professionalism versus unionism. The second is the views expressed about nursing by hospital management and the medical profession and the attempts of these groups to control nursing matters. These issues are not separate from the themes of domination and liberation. Both issues and themes are intertwined with each other, serving as factors of cause and effect which I shall attempt to illustrate with some historical data.

PROFESSIONALISM VERSUS UNIONISM IN NURSING

To give perspective on the issue of professionalism versus unionism, we need to clarify in our minds what professionalism is as a social phenomenon. For purposes of doing this, let us look at professionalism from a sociological approach which "views a profession as an organized group which is constantly interacting with the society that forms its matrix, which performs its social functions through a network of formal and informal relationships, and which creates its own subculture requiring adjustments to it as a prerequisite for career success."[3]

From its earliest days, organized nursing in every way met the terms of this definition of what it meant to be a profession. Nursing, along with medicine and dentistry, was one of the first three organized professions in the health field. Our two major professional "societies" or associations were officially formed between 1890 and 1900. At that time, no one except male members of the medical profession publicly opposed or seriously questioned nursing's right to claim professional status. Our profession was *the nursing profession.* Both then and now, we were and are the only nursing profession the American society has ever had. Moreover, regardless of how our profession may change its form and structure, we will continue to be the only profession qualified to provide essential nursing services to the public.

As nurses, we all know that our professional status has been attacked and questioned for a century. This castigation and belittlement of us has been a matter of social injustice and prejudice. The social injustices nurses have had to contend with over time did not in any way alter the fact of our existence as the nursing profession. The major effect of these injustices has been that of giving rise to our second-class status as opposed to our having a first-class status as professionals.

I want this point to be clearly understood for one main reason: It is extremely important in any discussion of the issue of professionalism versus unionism in nursing. The fact that we are a professional group which has traditionally labored with our hands resulted in the attachment of a stigma to nursing work. Historically, the "dignity" of our human labor has been put-down by powerful groups because of the manual labor involved in nursing work. Our knowledge and the use of our minds has received much less attention than has the use of our hands.

The very issue of professionalism versus unionism in nursing grew out of the fact that nurses were exploited because of the economic value of what they produced with their hands. From the nineteenth century on, the hours of labor extracted from nurses paralleled those of laboring men. And in truth, nurses were forced to work longer hours than most laboring men. Although this condition applied to both graduate nurses and to student nurses, the exploitation of student labor was the first to arouse public controversy over poor working conditions in nursing.

In 1896, Mary Adelaide Nutting, a prominent nursing leader, compared the working hours of student nurses to those of laboring men:

> It may be said that from 56 to 60 hours a week are generally considered fair working hours for the laboring man . . . few industries require their employees to work more than 10 hours daily and their Sundays are usually free. . . . We cannot actually compare industries with training schools . . . but we can state that a pupil in a training school may work harder to receive her training than a laboring man to support his wife and family, for here we find in one of the most difficult and responsible careers a woman can undertake, that her only method of receiving a certain kind of education is not to work 60 hours a week, but a number of hours varying from that number to 105.[4]

Nursing's association with labor came into being despite our professional organizations, despite our codes of ethics, and despite the self-identification of nurses as professionals. This association with labor merely reflected realities existing in practice settings where hospital management was in control of working conditions. Our professional associations were relatively powerless, having little or no say or authority over conditions of work in nursing. The unfair exploitation of nursing as a labor force began in the very decade that our profession was officially organized. The custom or tradition of working nurses 60 to 105 hours a week was a reality throughout the country, in every state prior to the date of 1913.

Though the overworking of nurses was unjust, hospital management evidenced no concern for justice, nor did hospitals express any real concern for the professional growth and development of young women in nursing. Both the health of nurses and their personal and professional growth were considered of secondary importance to hospital management. Nurses provided cheap labor not unlike that of "slave" labor and it was this labor that kept hospitals operating efficiently. Nurses, whether students or graduates, were considered dispensable persons; if one became ill or died from overwork, no one really cared because another graduate or student could be easily recruited to replace any nurse who could not tolerate the rigors of manual labor so highly valued by hospital management.

If you do not already know this, you will be most proud and perhaps pleased to learn that the citizens and nurse practitioners in your own state of California were the very first to make a public and open issue out of the unethical practices surrounding poor and unfair conditions of work within nursing. California was the first state in the nation to enact legislation controlling the exploitation and abuse of student nurse labor within hospitals.

In 1913, hospitals in California were defined by law as "continuous industries" and as such these institutions were forced to limit the working hours of women to eight a day.[5] This was the first protective law passed in the country which recognized the abuse of nurses by management. The passage of this law created a nationwide controversy in the health field which lasted for well over a decade. The influence of this legislation is still operative because the three eight-hour shifts now observed in hospitals across the country became the pattern of staffing as an outgrowth of legal reforms in California. Prior to that time, most hospitals observed some variation of two shifts with nurses working from 12 to 16 hours a day.

The controversy engendered by this 1913 legal reform is far more complicated than I can possibly explain in this paper today. My main reason for making reference to it is that the reform was brought about by the sponsorship and leadership of members of the California State Bureau of Labor. Also, although this was a good and necessary legal advancement for the nursing profession, it was not recognized as such by some leading nurses at the time. Nursing was very much divided then on the issue of professionalism versus unionism and the involvement of labor in support of nursing legislation disturbed a lot of nurses. The California Nurses' Association opposed the bill; nursing service administrators and directors opposed the bill. Hospital management opposed the bill, and the medical profession came out in opposition to it.

This needed social reform became a reality because of the support of nurse practitioners, the support of citizen groups, and because of the support of organized labor. Though opposing improvements in both nursing education and practice, nurses who identified with hospital management did not support nursing but took the side of hospital management on this issue. Repressive politics were surely operative then as now within hospital settings.

The CNA did not support this social reform in nursing because the bill was sponsored by the State Department of Labor. Nursing leaders connected with CNA resented the intrusion of labor into the affairs of nursing because the interest of organized labor in nursing was perceived as a threat to the professional image and "dignity" of the nursing profession. Moreover, the CNA did not want to be publicly identified as a "labor pressure group." Leading nurses within the CNA were not opposed to improving working conditions in hospitals, they merely wanted to achieve reforms in a more "dignified manner" through the efforts of the professional association and its nurse practice act and not through the support of labor.[6]

The position of CNA is quite understandable since the stigma attached to the stereotype of labor in the American society was something to be avoided. The fear of having this stigma attached to nursing work blinded nursing leaders to the fact that they were in reality a professional group of laboring people with a second-class status already, both as working women and as professionals. Nurses representing CNA did not, and rightfully so, want to be classified as "trade unionists" at the time. These nurses did, however, underestimate the power of their opposition and did not realize that the nurse practice acts would never cut down on the abuses directed toward nurses in practice settings.

Hospital management in California was so adamantly opposed to the eight-hour law passed in 1913 that they put forth organized efforts to have the law repealed. In 1915, the case went to the Supreme Court of the United States. Hospitals claimed that restricting the hours of work of nurses was "unconstitutional" violating the hospitals' "freedom of contract."[7] As nurses, we can be thankful for those good citizens serving on the Supreme Court then because representatives of hospital management lost the case. The Court ruled that the law was indeed constitutional. The whole issue was a question of social justice and the court's decision was an attempt to curtail the commercial abuse of nurses, at least in the state of California.

Despite this final court decision, prominent individuals in management continued to protest that the law was unconstitutional and even unhumanitarian. For example, in 1915 shortly after the Supreme Court had acted, Dr. H. T. Summergill, Superintendent of the University of California Hospital and then president of the American Hospital Association, told members of that association: "On its face . . . [the bill regulating hospitals] appears to be contrary to the principles of not only the American Constitution but to all principles of humanity."[8]

Obviously the humanity of nurses and their rights meant nothing to this physician and hospital administrator. In his view the California law was itself inhumane, but the continuing exploitation of young women for the economic gain of hospitals was not. This view was a commonly held one throughout the country. Nursing was destined to suffer much from similar views on the part of physicians and hospital administrators.

During the second and third decades of this century, the issue of professionalism versus unionism was heatedly debated all over this country in cities and in small towns. It was a national issue in the health field. In an editorial appearing in *The Modern Hospital*, the editor noted that "the time will never come when the professional woman shall cease to feel the stigma of legislation secured through the efforts of labor, however well intended such efforts may have been."[9] This editor had little vision about the future because we are now living at a time when the professional woman or man need not feel any stigma whatever by resorting to the use of labor or any other group in efforts to improve their lot in life.

However, back when the California law was passed, the times were different. The worst fears of the CNA did come to pass. Increasingly, nurses were not only labeled "trade unionists", they were also designated as a group that was "undemocratic," "un-American," and "class oriented."[10] These false and demeaning terms were directed toward nurses all because they were trying to preserve their human dignity as a professional group having both the obligation and the right to improve their status. These unkind labels came from both hospital management and from propaganda dispensed by groups of physicians throughout the country.

Greatly concerned about the issue of professionalism versus unionism, Anna C. Jamme of the CNA wrote to Mary Adelaide Nutting of New York City about the problems of nurses in California. Nutting responded to her letter saying:

> I am really not a bit worried about the dignity of the profession of nursing. . . . It is entirely true as your legislators state, that nurses everywhere are overworked and underpaid. Among those who believe in the true dignity of labor, we should rank high and not feel that anything but good can come of the efforts of labor organizations to help those who labor.[11]

Jamme must have been a most conscientious and good-hearted nurse because she continued to worry about the nursing profession and its dignity. She wrote Nutting several times. Nutting stressed her strong views on the beneficial efforts of labor organizations in helping to improve conditions for workers in hospitals:

The hours of work now required of pupil nurses and graduate nurses in hospitals and out of them, are oppressive, a menace to the health of the workers, and indirectly . . . to the health and welfare of those for whom they care . . . if the philanthropists and others throughout our country . . . will not come to the aid of those who labor it is time for labor to step in and control the matter. I see no real loss of dignity in so doing; yet I know how you all feel, that in some way the dignity of our profession will be impaired and the status of nursing lowered, and I wish it were possible to secure righteous conditions . . . in other ways. Experience covering half a century and over, appears to show that this is difficult if not impossible of accomplishment.[12]

Many nursing practitioners in California must have felt much the same way as Nutting on the question of social justice for nurses and on the issue of professionalism versus unionism for it was their support as nurses and as politically active citizens that served to bring about a significant legal reform. One California nurse, Marie Hadden, viewed the whole affair as a "spectacle" since "*all* hospital authorities, most training school superintendents and the medical profession" in California were "clamoring for the repeal of a law, the need of such law having been so clearly shown."[13]

I hope we nurses today can learn something from these historical examples of past behavior on the part of significant persons in the health field as they reacted to issues related to nursing. With the exception of studying the problem further and being fully informed as to its meaning for us as professionals, we nurses today need to bury the issue of professionalism versus unionism. As we can learn from the past, our dignity as a profession is not at stake now and it never really has been at stake. We have only thought it was and have, as a result, conformed to much that could do nothing to advance our cause.

With management in control of nursing in practice settings, our problems have remained those of labor and management. The need for collective bargaining today is an outgrowth of this historical situation. For a century, in the minds of both hospital management and physicians, nurses have had no real professional status or "dignity" to be maintained. Cast in the unsavory role of menial labor, our rights as professionals have been denied us. Both hospital administration and the medical profession have been more powerful than nursing and the views of the more powerful have prevailed. Keeping nursing in a subservient role has been to their advantage. This role has not been to the advantage of us nurses, and it has not been to the advantage of patients, nor has it been beneficial to the cause of improving quality in health care.

Medical and Hospital Domination of Nurses: Social Discrimination

To more fully illustrate the nature of some real problems facing us nurses today, I want to give you some more historical data to provide proof of the extent to which we have been dominated by groups more powerful than us. The following data explains some of the root causes of blatant social discrimination directed toward nurses and toward our profession. This data can further explain why we have been repeatedly cast in the role of labor and why we nurses have worried so about our "dignity" as a profession.

As a result of social injustices directed toward us, we nurses have simply not enjoyed the fruits and rewards of living in a democracy. Too many limitations have been placed on our thinking and on our behavior. Both external and internal limitations of a social and psychological nature have prevented our progress in more ways than one. Dominant groups have superimposed these limitations upon us, and it is high time we actively take it upon ourselves to correct the situation before another wasted decade passes.

To give perspective on the nature of domination we have been subjected to, nurses were historically treated as if they were objects to be used and abused, and not human beings with dignity, worthy of respect and support equal to that provided other groups in the health field. Keeping nurses in an inferior and limited position was repeatedly urged in medical literature. The following statement from the *Journal of the American Medical Association* clearly illustrates continuing efforts to dominate and to restrict the actions of nurses:

Every attempt at initiative on the part of nurses . . . should be re-proved by the physician and by the hospital administration. 2. The programs of nursing schools . . . should be limited strictly to the in-dispensable matters of instruction for those in their position. . . . The professional instruction of . . . nurses should be entrusted exclusively to the physicians who only can judge what is necessary for them to know.[14]

Keeping the nurse in her "proper sphere" and in her limited "province" was declared to be the duty of both the physician and the hospital administrator. Physicians, in particular, repeatedly argued that nurses

. . . should cultivate a pleasant temper, cheerful countenance and encouraging demeanor. . . . She should . . . never attempt to appear learned and of great importance. . . . In addition to these funda-mental essentials, she should be able and willing to render . . . obe-dience to the instructions of the attending physician and carry out his orders to the letter.[15]

It was views such as these which surely motivated hospital officials to work young nurses for as many hours as 60 to 105 a week without re-gard for the health or well-being of the nurse as a person. Only some-one with an intense desire to dominate another human would want a person to behave in the manner described by the physician I just quoted. Another quote illustrates the intensity of the desire of medical men to rule over women in nursing and control them with an iron hand.

As medical men put it: "The education of the trained nurse for ob-vious reasons should be under the supervision of the medical profes-sion; and hospital nurse superintendents and head nurses *especially*, the subjects of intelligent official control."[16] Of notable significance, our leaders in key positions of nursing service directors and head nurses are referred to as "subjects." According to Webster's dictio-nary, a "subject" is "one that is placed under authority or control" or a subject is "one who lives within the territory of . . . and owes alle-giance to a sovereign power or state." Only a slave or a person in a very servile status is likely to be referred to and treated as a "subject" in need of constant and "official" control.

Since nurses in the hospital setting were treated as "subjects" by both physicians and hospital administrators, it is little wonder that the nurses in California who identified with hospital management came out in support of management instead of nursing back in 1913 when the eight-hour law was passed. Given the repressive circumstances in which they worked, these nurses were probably afraid they would lose their jobs if they did not support hospital management. The climates within which nurses work today are just as repressive as they were back in the first decade of this century. Efforts to dominate and control nurses are just as severe now as then.

As nurses, we must begin to carefully examine both the attitudes of physicians and hospital administrators. And we must encourage and urge the public to begin to do this also. The views these groups hold about nursing are very damaging to both nurses and to the public's welfare where health care is concerned. These powerful groups I have mentioned have perpetuated many misconceptions about nursing, and currently the public scarcely knows who nurses are or what we do.

To further illustrate some of the damaging views spread around about us, in the twenties, the president of the American Medical Association, in a speech at their national convention, emphasized that "the proper work of the trained nurse does not contemplate that she is in a position of primary responsibility. . . . The things she has to do are simple things."[17] It has been such statements as this one which has resulted in the brainwashing of the public about the superiority of the physician and the inferiority of the nurse.

"Subjects," slaves, and domestic servants have traditionally been considered "simple" souls and good-natured objects designed for use by others. Such "subjects" hardly needed to be educated for a professional role. In the thirties, this view of nurses is clearly expressed in the words of the president of the American Hospital Association who emphasized that nurses did not need higher education because to educate them was like educating "a people beyond their sphere of usefulness."[18] This particular physician and hospital administrator went further stressing the point that nurses should, he strongly believed, "enter the nursing profession for the love of the work and the good they may do."[19] This is ridiculous since we all know that in our society people work for pay not for love. Being paid for honest work is an American value we all hold dear, as women or as men.

I wish to emphasize here that it was physicians and hospital administrators who labeled nurses "trade unionists," "undemocratic," and "class oriented" when nurses were only fighting for their rights to better pay, to better working conditions, and for their rights to have their human dignity respected in the same manner in which the human dignity of other professional groups was respected. Physicians repeatedly demeaned nursing's professional associations by calling them "unions," a word they would not have used in making reference to the American Medical Association.[20]

Social discrimination and prejudice toward nurses and toward our profession has been perpetuated by the dominant organizations of the medical profession and of hospital administration over the century. The system of control fostered by them has not been democratic, but autocratic and dictatorial. In reality, nurses have had to contend with a form of policy and a decision-making process which has been more like a form of despotism than it has been representative of a democratic form of governance of affairs in nursing and in health care. Today, our generation of nurses needs to liberate the nursing profession from this type of despotic influence. The repressive politics being directed toward us nurses in every state is a manifestation of this despotic influence.

You may well question my judgment in using so strong a word as despotism. You may be thinking that nurses were to blame for their own suppression. You may be thinking to yourself by now that the severity of nursing's oppression was really the fault of nurses themselves who should have gotten over their differences of opinion and unified themselves into a group powerful enough to overcome the forces keeping them down. You will be quite right if you are thinking that nurses did consent to many of the wishes of those who oppressed them.

To support my own statement on despotism, I want to share with you a quote which can enlighten us on the nature of some of the consenting behavior nurses manifested in the past. Since oppression is always a complex political and social problem, let us think about political freedom for a moment. According to Alexander Meiklejohn, political freedom

> . . . cannot be understood unless we distinguish sharply and persistently between the "submission" of a slave and the "consent" of a free citizen. In both cases it is agreed that obedience shall be required. Even when despotism is so extreme as to be practically indistinguishable from enslavement, a pseudo consent is given by the subjects. When the ruling force is overwhelming, . . . (humans) are driven not only to submit, but also to agree to do so. For the time, at least, they decide to make the best of a bad situation rather than to struggle against hopeless odds. And, coordinate with this "submission" by the people, there are "concessions" by the ruler. For the avoiding of trouble, to establish his power, to manipulate one hostile force against another, he must take account of the desires and interests of his subjects, must manage to keep them from becoming too rebellious. The granting of such "concessions" and the accepting of them are, perhaps, the clearest evidence that a government is not democratic but is essentially despotic and alien.[21]

I repeat, what nurses dealt with historically and what we nurses are dealing with now are forces that operate more in a despotic fashion than in a democratic one. Given such a situation as this, the need to increase our power to overcome such dominant forces is quite evident. Another quote is useful here to clarify the meaning of power where despotic influences are concerned:

> When one man or some self-chosen group holds control, without full consent, over others, the relation between them is one of force and counterforce, of compulsion on the one hand and submission or resistance on the other. . . . The only basic fact is that one group "has the power" and the other group or groups do not. In such a despotism, a ruler, by some excess of strength, guile or both without the consent of his subjects, forces them into obedience. And in order to understand what he does, what they do, we need only

measure the strength or weakness of the control and the strength or weakness of the resistance to it.[22]

In comparison to the combined power of medicine and hospital administration, we nurses have scarcely been strong. Hospital administration, moreover, has never willingly made any outstanding "concessions" to nurses. Thus, the support of both labor and groups of citizens was necessary to force hospitals to cut the working hours of student nurses to a decent eight-hour day; and as we saw from what happened right here in California in 1913, hospitals protested this just measure of reform by denying the need for any legal reforms to improve conditions in nursing. We still today need the support of labor and of various groups of citizens to bring about reforms in the health care system and in nursing.

The year 1976 is just around the corner. As a profession half as old as this country itself, we should enter 1976 with the spirit of reform flowing throughout our veins. With or without complete and full unity as a profession, nurses in towns and cities all over this country should seek to improve their status in all communities. Organized efforts at the local level are just as important as political and social action at the national and state levels. In truth, organized action at a local level may well be more important than other kinds because nurses work in local communities in various types of social institutions, and it is the latter that we must change. Power at the local level will be the key to achieving power at the national level.

As I mentioned earlier, we nurses need to try to understand and respect each other more. As a profession we have tremendous potential to improve health care in this country and this should be our major priority and goal in the year of 1976. Our profession has served this nation for over a century without much public recognition or support for the contributions we make in health care. We have, therefore, labored under severe handicaps. It is time we received more respect, more benefits, more pay, more professional privileges, and more freedom to act in providing comprehensive nursing services to all that need this service.

The first step toward health care reforms is that of getting the burden of oppression off the backs of nurses now. The chains of the past we must break. Quality in health care depends upon the freedom of nurses to provide it, and we cannot serve the public well while our rights to freedom and support are being denied to us. In reflecting upon the slow advancement of nursing, we should all think about a comment once made by Mary Adelaide Nutting:

> Well may . . . [nursing] say as Christian, in the Pilgrim's Progress, said to Pliable who urged him to mend his pace—"I cannot go as fast as I would by reason of this burden which is on my back."[23]

Though she did not call it what it was, this outstanding nursing historian, teacher, and leader was talking about the burden of oppression on the back of her profession and our profession. We nurses of today can do what the nurses of the past could not do; we can acquire the power necessary for achieving our liberation from dominant powers that have treated us unjustly. As we work toward this goal, we will eventually have a sense of unity too as a profession whose services are absolutely essential to any kind of quality in health care.

Our common cause is that of fighting for social justice. Achieving social justice and our equality with other professional groups can lead to a kind of unification we nurses have never known before. The power to do this resides in each of us regardless of which state we live in or where we may work. In a spirit of persistence and determination, let us make 1976 the best and most exciting year we nurses have ever had. Let us this coming year take our case to the public for our cause is their cause too. Quality in health care does not depend upon medicine. It depends upon the freedom of nurses to provide quality in nursing. As a profession, we owe physicians nothing, and we owe hospitals nothing, but we do owe American citizens a great deal as guardians of their health.

REFERENCES

1. Freire, P. (1972). *Pedagogy of the oppressed* (p. 93). New York: Herder and Herder.

2. Williams, W. A. (1961). *The contours of American history* (p. 479). Chicago: Quadrangle Books.

3. Vollmer, H. M., & Mills, D. L. (Eds.). (1966). *Professionalization* (p. 10). Englewood Cliffs, NJ: Prentice-Hall, Inc.

4. Nutting, M. A. (1896). "A Statistical Report of Working Hours in Training Schools." *Proceedings of the American society of superintendents of training schools*, 36.

5. Anna C. Jamme to Mary Adelaide Nutting, 1 May 1913, Nutting Papers, Archives of the Department of Nursing Education, Teachers College, Columbia University, New York, New York. (All subsequent letters cited are located in these Archives.) See also, *Proceedings of the N.L.N.E.*, 1913, p. 79.

6. Jamme to Nutting, 1 May 1913.

7. *Transactions of the American Hospital Association*, 1915, p. 130.

8. *Ibid.*, p. 91.

9. "Editorial," *The Modern Hospital*, Vol. 2 (1914, April), p. 260.

10. See The *Nurse*, Vol. 1 (1921, February), p. 7; also, Vol. 2 (1921, September), pp. 5–6.

11. Nutting to Jamme, 9 May 1913.

12. Nutting to Jamme, 3 May 1913.

13. Marie Hadden to Nutting, 11 October 1913.

14. "Nurses' Schools and Illegal Practice of Medicine," *The Journal of the American Medical Association*, Vol. 47 (December 1, 1906), p. 1835.

15. Beates, H. (1909). *The status of nurses: A sociologic problem* (p. 7). Philadelphia: Physicians' National Board of Regents.

16. *Ibid.*, p. 21.

17. Pusey, W. A. (1924, June 14). "The Trend in Medical and Nursing Services." *The Journal of the American Medical Association*, Vol. 82, 1961.

18. *Transactions of the American Hospital Association*, 1931, p. 196.

19. *Ibid.*, p. 197.

20. Mayo, W. (1920, July 31). "Observations on South America." *The Journal of the American Medical Association*, Vol. 75, 314.

21. Meiklejohn, A. (1965). *Political freedom: The constitutional powers of the people* (pp. 14–15). New York: Oxford University Press.

22. *Ibid.*, p. 11.

23. Nutting, M. A. (1921, March). "Again the Call to Duty." *American Journal of Nursing*, Vol. 21, 364.

Chapter 7

PROFESSIONALISM AND THE LAW

INTRODUCTORY COMMENTS

*I*nternational Women's Year has come and gone. As women, we must ask ourselves if this past year and its events brought women of the world any closer together as people and as persons. A year's focus on the problems and concerns of women is nothing in comparison to the centuries women have lived, lived often in misery and in poverty. Nurses all over the world need to begin an unending international movement to foster the improvement of women's health. Women's health problems are surely much the same the world over, regardless of their race, creed, or nationality.

At this point in the history of the world, the world has grown small. We are all neighbors dealing with similar economic, political, and social problems. Moreover, we are presently living in sad times, times that make our economic, political, and social problems more complex than we might want them to be. We are living in bad times. Our value systems are in a state of change with cultural revolutions in the making. Changes such as these always give rise to bad times for living humans. All over the world, in country after country, human misery, human terror rules and reigns in the hearts and minds of large segments of humanity.

Lecture presented at the Festival of Life and Learning Program, sponsored by the School of Nursing, University of Manitoba, Manitoba, Canada, February 4, 1977.

Dominant controls and societal forces continue to keep various peoples oppressed and depressed. As a result, people everywhere have health problems staring them in the face daily. Hugging their misery close, people all over the world are searching for ways to escape their misery; at the same time, many are searching for ways to enlarge their humanness.

The spiritual character of humanity is in desperate need of a festival renewal. Your own Festival of Life and Learning is surely a manifestation of this need to renew life and the forces that can keep a life healthy. In my own country, the decay in human spirits is a major health problem. The laws of our land foster this decay in numerous ways. The laws, for example, have helped to turn our health care system into a disease oriented system that places little emphasis on health. In our capitalistic system, profits are made off of keeping people unhealthy, profits are made especially from women who comprise the largest group seeking help from disease oriented professionals. In addition to being harmful to the health of women generally, our laws support systems that kill the spirits of nurses preventing them from providing the health care they are educated and trained to provide.

THE UNHEALTHY PHENOMENA OF SPLITTING HUMANS INTO COMPARTMENTS

Before elaborating specifically upon professionalism and the law, I want to comment on a basic problem related to scientific developments and medical technology. With the advancement of science and medical technology, our society has split the human being into fragmented compartments. This is a predicament far, far removed from the ideal of human wholeness, a concept and condition essential for the emergence of human health. Humans are not pieces of furniture to be repaired and polished. They are not machines with parts to be fixed, greased, or manipulated. Humans have a body, mind, and soul. The health of body and mind go hand in hand to make a healthy whole person. The wholistically integrated human being can withstand many a storm in life.

However, in contrast, splitting the human into parts gives rise to misery and to disease. For health to come this splitting of persons must stop.

The splitting of humans into conflicting parts goes well beyond the realm of patient care as reflected in the fragmented services provided by specialists. The splitting of humans is also reflected in our divisions of labor. To examine the phenomena of splitting humans into compartments, we can analyze the diverse influences impinging upon the role of the nursing profession within health care delivery systems and within society.

As we all know, any social order has laws defining and giving shape and form to that social order. Divisions of labor and professional functioning are supposedly controlled by laws. Passing laws is an attempt to control human behavior setting boundaries and limits that may or may not be transcended by the actions of humans. Where professions are concerned, the laws can define, limit, or restrict the extent to which a group can achieve high levels of professional conduct. Laws can give freedom to act or they can restrict freedom preventing certain actions. Within the health field, laws have given unlimited freedom of action to the profession of medicine; while doing this, similar laws regulating nursing practice have been restricting to the freedom and actions of practitioners in this field. Laws quite frequently determine the nature of relationships in the world of human action. The latter has certainly been the case where nursing's relationships to medicine, hospitals, and clients are concerned.

In any given society, it is not uncommon to find conflicts and contradictions between what the law says and what goes on in the world of reality and action. In other words, laws are written to control human behavior but human behavior often defies the law or differs from what the law states. Thus, laws become outdated and ineffective, and must be changed as the times call for this. In a book entitled *The Human Condition*, Hannah Arendt comments upon the limitations of law and human institutions:

> Limitations and boundaries exist within the realm of human affairs, but they never offer a framework that can reliably withstand

the onslaught with which each new generation must insert itself. The frailty of human institutions and laws and, generally, of all matters pertaining to men's living together, arises from the human condition of natality and is quite independent of the frailty of human nature . . . the territorial boundaries which protect and make possible the physical identity of a people, and the laws which protect and make possible its political existence, are of such great importance to the stability of human affairs precisely because no such limiting and protecting principles rise out of the activities going on in the realm of human affairs itself. The limitations of the law are never entirely reliable safeguards against action from within the body politic, just as the boundaries of the territory are never entirely reliable safeguards against action from without. The boundlessness of action is only the other side of its tremendous capacity for establishing relationships, that is, its specific productivity; this is why the old virtue of moderation, of keeping within bounds, is indeed one of the political virtues par excellence . . .[1]

Hannah Arendt is making some very important observations about human behavior, laws, and institutions. She emphasizes that limitations and boundaries are not useful frameworks when social change is in order. This observation is fascinating when applied to law and professionalism in nursing. Where nursing is concerned, a framework of limitations and boundaries has been operative for over a century now. However inappropriate, this has been so because nurses have been predominantly women. The logic has been that because nurses were women limitations and boundaries had to be placed on their behaviors and actions. Our laws have been written accordingly, restricting nurses rather than liberating them to function as fully qualified professionals with accompanying privileges and rewards. Our laws reflect more about our role as women than they do about our role as professionals. The boundaries and limitations constricting our functions in society have actually resulted in our being denied professional status equal to men in professions.

Our generation of nurses must question the use of a framework of limitations and boundaries when applied to our physical and professional identity. Our laws must be re-written with another framework in mind, a framework that defines us as professionals and not just licensed workers who must be employed by agencies repressing our actions and our freedom in giving society the nursing care it needs. Presently and in the future, the territory we carve out for ourselves should reflect no restrictions on nursing's professional capacity to provide wholistic care to the publics we serve.

Let me go a step further to elaborate upon contradictions and conflicts inherent in laws and social institutions as these are related to human behavior and action. Nurses are educated as professionals. Nurses are licensed by law as professionals. And yet these same laws often state that nurses must be supervised by a licensed physician. This is an obvious contradiction where the meaning of professional action is concerned. Another contradiction arises and lies in the fact that although nurses are educated as professionals they are in practice settings employed and treated as mere workers. The professional identity crisis nurses have talked about for years grows directly out of these contradictions.

The damaging effects of these contradictions can be observed in the lives of young women and men who enter the nursing profession. The splitting phenomena I talked about earlier affects all nurses. Psychologically and in the physical world of work, the young nurse practitioner today is split into splinters soon after graduation. To illustrate this point, I will share with you a quote from a letter I recently received from a practitioner prepared to function as a professional, and eager to grow more and more professional with experience. She wrote,

> I am young, relatively apolitical, and certainly naive in many respects—yet I can perceive the disparity that exists in society, in health care, in the power structures of both! . . . change is imperative, and . . . I must be a part of such change. I am overwhelmed by the task, frustrated by my own powerlessness and the ignorance and apathy of my peers. I have been a practitioner for just about five months now, and though I suffer from reality shock . . . I can objectively identify the inherent problems in the system—no collective bargaining for nurses, incompetent nurses in supervisory

positions . . . the research disease orientation of the physicians. While I'm struggling to establish a professional self identity, the system sees me as a licensed worker. This question of the dual role as professional and employee is a new one for me—one that I must explore. While it is easy to be cynical, I am trying not to be.[2]

This young practitioner is suffering from the outcomes and consequences growing out of gross contradictions inherent in laws and the functioning of societal institutions. Social institutions, such as hospitals, are in no way legally forced to respect the rights of nurses. As far as professional nurses are concerned these social agencies do not view the nurses as having rights at all. Throughout the United States, for example, nurses are engaged in legal struggles to win their rights to earn their daily bread. Nurses must strike to obtain rights. And, in many states it is illegal for nurses to strike. When nurses do strike to obtain meager rights, they are abused by society and the laws too. The laws we have written on the books today in no way protect nurses; instead, they permit various agencies to legally abuse nurses.

To illustrate the inhumane nature of this legal abuse, nurses in Chicago, Illinois, recently went on strike. They did so in an attempt to force hospitals to give them a reasonable deal where sick pay is concerned. In Illinois, the law says that public employees may not legally strike. However, with hospitals refusing to grant sick pay or to give sick days to the nurses, the nurses decided to break the law, striking illegally for their cause which was a higher cause than the cause of the law. The Illinois Nurses' Association attempted to support the nurses in their strike, but the courts immediately fined the Association $1,000.00 for this supportive action. The courts further specified that the amount of this fine would increase to the tune of $10,000.00 a day for any additional days of support given by the Association. Thus, the law not only condoned the hospital's abuse of nurses, it also prevented organized nursing from supporting practitioners in nursing. This is a clear-cut example of the splitting phenomena—in this case, operating to destroy any kind of unity nurses might have been able to maintain in achieving their aims for better working conditions.

In this situation, no one except the nurses questioned the inhumaneness of the Health and Hospitals Governing Commission's position that nurses should receive "no pay for the first day of illness until a nurse . . . (had) been working at the hospitals for three years."[3] In taking this position, hospital officials clearly indicate their lack of respect for nurses. Contending constantly with such attitudes of disrespect, nurses are not treated as humans let alone as professionals. Our laws support and give legal sanction to this type of inhumane treatment of nurses.

Legal repression and abuse of nurses is a pervasive problem in the United States. This repression is not a new problem; it is as old as the profession itself. The question of law and order in a society is a political and an economic question. The problem of repression is also a political and an economic one. The legal boundaries and limitations placed upon nurses are really placed there for economic and political reasons. The economic status of nurses prevents nurses from changing many a law that needs changing this day and age.

THE ECONOMIC POSITION OF WOMEN: THE CONCEPT OF THE CONVENIENT SOCIAL VIRTUE

The economic status of nurses and of women in society are one and the same. John Kenneth Galbraith very astutely describes the debilitated role of women in our American society. As Galbraith puts it:

> The search for surrogates has led generally to women and the family. It has made use of a pervasive force in the shaping of social attitudes—one that has often been sensed but rarely described. A name for it is needed, and it may be called the Convenient Social Virtue.
>
> The convenient social virtue ascribes merit to any pattern of behavior, however uncomfortable or unnatural for the individual involved, that serves the comfort or well-being of, or is otherwise advantageous for, the more powerful members of the community. The moral commendation of the community for convenient and therefore virtuous behavior then serves as a substitute for pecuniary (monetary) compensation. Inconvenient behavior becomes

deviant behavior and is subject to the righteous disapproval or sanction of the community.

The convenient social virtue is widely important for inducing people to perform unpleasant services. . . . Anyone resistant to such service was condemned as deeply unpatriotic or otherwise despicable. The convenient social virtue has also helped obtain the charitable and compassionate services of nurses, custodial personnel and other hospital staff. Here too the resulting merit in the eyes of the community served as a partial substitute for compensation. (Such merit was never deemed a wholly satisfactory substitute for remuneration in the case of physicians.) Numerous other tasks for the public good—those commonly characterized as charitable works—are also greatly reduced in cost by the convenient social virtue. But the convenient social virtue has been most useful of all in solving the problem of menial personal service. . . . The ultimate success of the convenient social virtue has been in converting women to menial personal service.[4]

Galbraith's main point is this: "the labor of women to facilitate consumption is not valued in national income or product."[5] First and foremost, he describes women as dependent parasites playing out a quasi-servant role essential to the maintenance of economic structures as we know them now. In this role, the lives of women can have no meaning unless they are attached to the lives of people more powerful than they are, people who use women as objects to meet their own ends. Our laws and our socialization processes re-enforce the need for women to attach themselves to the more powerful.

The role of the housewife is not unlike the menial role assumed by nurses or domestic labor generally. Galbraith explains this menial role,

The conversion of women into a crypto-servant class was an economic accomplishment of the first importance. Menially employed servants were available only to a minority of the preindustrial population; the servant-wife is available, democratically, to almost the entire present male population. . . . The servant role of women is critical for the expansion of consumption in the modern economy.

That it is so generally approved . . . is a formidable tribute to the power of the convenient social virtue.[6]

Keeping women in parasitical servant roles or locking them into low-paid service positions naturally gives rise to all kinds of health and illness problems on the part of women. Women's consumption of disease oriented care can keep physicians and hospitals in business. From data gathered while doing health work with low-income women, I am convinced that the major cause of women's health problems derives from their being socialized to believe their happiness and sense of well-being resides outside themselves. As the result of living out pre-defined social roles, the vast majority of women spend their lives seeking relationships that foster their dependency in child-like roles, not their healthy liberation as self-sufficient beings.

Dependency relationships, such as marriage for example, offer far more advantages to men than to women. Statistics reveal that marriage for women can be a health hazard. As the author of *Passages* points out,

> . . . the mental health hazards suffered by married women are far greater than those of married men. Sociologist Jessie Bernard has brought to light startling evidence on this score. More married women than married men have felt they were about to have a nervous breakdown; more have experienced psychological and physical anxiety; more have had feelings of inadequacy in their marriages and blamed themselves for their passivity, and mental health impairment.[7]

I have used this material on the mental health problems of married women for one main reason. The relationships nurses have to maintain with physicians and with hospitals employing them are very much like the dependency relationships women form in marriages. Our laws have, of course, always forced these roles upon nurses. Just as the livelihood of the wife is dependent upon her attachment to a husband, the livelihood of the nurses is dependent upon their attachment to doctors or to hospitals. This goes back to the old notion that women, in order to obtain economic support, happiness, and wholeness, must attach themselves to someone more powerful than they are. Where nurses are concerned, this has many political, economic, and legal ramifications.

Weak from a political standpoint, nurses have been slow to examine their attachments to institutions or to other individuals they work with daily. Many of these attachments actually prevent nurses from practicing nursing as it should be practiced. For example, because of our unhealthy attachments to others, third-party reimbursement for nursing practice outside of a hospital is not a reality on any widespread scale; and even when provided, the physician must still be involved whether his services are needed or not. Though highly qualified as professionals nurses cannot earn a living being paid directly for the nursing services they can provide.

We need to change our laws so that nurses can truly function as professionals and be paid for their services directly without recourse to physicians or hospitals. The troublesome relationships nurses have to deal with in their practice are not conducive to maintaining the health of nurses. Although we do not have much research on the mental health hazards of becoming a nurse, I am sure data would reveal problems similar to those observed in married women. The anxieties and fears of nurses in the work setting and out of it are surely just as great. This is an area of concern needing to be thoroughly researched. Data along these lines could be useful in supporting the need for changing laws that are harmful to the health of nurses and to the health of patients as well.

LAW AND LEVELS OF PRACTICE IN NURSING: CLASS STRUGGLES MUST GO

I hope I have clarified some of the major considerations involved in the relationship between law and professionalism. At this point, I want to discuss the law and the levels of practice in nursing. Due to the nature of nursing's historical development, we are a far more complex profession than most. At this stage in our historical development, it is extremely important for all nurses to have a greater understanding of law and the nature of relationships between the various levels of practice within nursing itself. Non-professionals within nursing are just as important as the professionals and it is time nurses dealt with this issue in a more sane, humane, and wise fashion. The welfare and well-being of non-professionals in our field should be of prime concern to every professionally prepared nurse.

As all of you must know by now, in the hierarchy of the so-called health care system the whole of the nursing profession (professionals and non-professionals alike) are lumped into the same category. We are the persons with the lowest status. We are mostly women. We are the lowest paid. We are the laboring class, the working class. If nurses are to have a major impact on changing laws and the health care system, levels within nursing must achieve some sense of unity instead of the disunity and conflicts so often manifested in the relationships of professionals and non-professionals within the profession.

Let me say here, the theories of Karl Marx are most relevant to an understanding of the behavior of various levels of workers in nursing. It was Karl Marx who came up with the wonderful insight that all of history is a history of class struggles. It is Karl Marx who devoted his life and his research activity in efforts to free oppressed working classes from the miseries of capitalist domination. Since all nurses have historically been cast into the role of the subordinate working class or productive force within health care settings, a Marxist interpretation of our struggles and difficulties is imperative for providing new knowledge about and understanding of our plight in the world of work.

The historian, William Appleman Williams, in his book *The Great Evasion,* makes the point that Americans at a very high cost to themselves have ignored the theories of Marx. In the words of Williams,

Americans have never confronted Karl Marx himself. We have never confronted his central theses about the assumptions, the costs, and the nature of capitalist society. We have never confronted his central insight that capitalism is predicated upon an overemphasis and exaltation of the individualistic, egoistic half of man functioning in a marketplace system that overrides and crushes the social, humanitarian half of man. We have never confronted his perception that capitalism is based upon a definition of man in the marketplace that defines the dialogue between men as a competitive struggle for riches and power. And we have never confronted his argument that capitalism cannot create a community in which how much men produce and own is less important than what they make, less important than their relationships as they produce and distribute those products, less important than what they are as men, and less important than how they treat each other.[8]

With laws supporting a disease-oriented health care system causing almost more problems than it cures these days, we must take Marx seriously, doing historical, economic, and legal studies that will explain the damage done to humanity by this capitalistic system. For one sure thing, this system has certainly kept nurses oppressed and has nearly crushed our persons and all levels of our practice to death.

Let me share with you some of Marx's own thoughts which are so explanatory of the historical development of the levels of practice within the nursing profession. Marx wrote,

The history of all hitherto existing society is the history of class struggles.

Freeman and slave, patrician and plebeian, lord and serf, guildmaster and journeyman, in a word, oppressor and oppressed, stood in constant opposition to one another, carried on an uninterrupted, now hidden, now open fight, a fight that each time ended, either in a revolutionary reconstitution of society at large, or in the common ruin of the struggling classes.

In the earlier epochs of history, we find almost everywhere a complicated arrangement of society into various orders, a manifold gradation of social rank. In ancient Rome we have patricians, knights, plebeians, slaves; in the Middle Ages, feudal lords, vassals, guildmasters, journeymen, apprentices, serfs; and in almost all of these particular classes, again, other subordinate gradations.

The modern bourgeois society that has sprouted from the ruins of feudal society has not done away with class antagonisms. It has only established new classes, new conditions of oppression, new forms of struggle in place of the old ones.[9]

This Marxist analysis of classes describes the situation we have in our American health care system almost perfectly. Within the nursing profession itself the various groups or levels of practitioners behave as if they were separate classes, classes constantly struggling and fighting with each other as though in competition with each other for a place in society and in the marketplace. You are all familiar with the social and legal rankings within nursing: we have aides, licensed practical nurses, associate degree graduates, hospital diploma school graduates; we have baccalaureate degree graduates, all in a somewhat confused state about just who they are in relation to other workers.

At one point in our recent history this list of rankings read a bit differently: attendants, sub-nurses (short course and correspondence school graduates), apprentices, and the hospital graduate all in competition for economic rewards from the practice of nursing. The class struggles and the competition between these various rankings presented numerous problems which the laws and our legal system generally did nothing about. Historically, the laws did not protect nurses; and, they did not protect the public from the same types of abuse and exploitation the nurses were subjected to in the health field.

Today as in the past, the laws regulating the administration of any delivery of health and medical care do not protect the people who give this care. And, it is common knowledge that the law has not and does not control scandals, fraud, and the exploitation of the public where health care services are concerned. This ineffectiveness of the law means one thing: there is a drastic need for changing many, many laws regulating the health care system and the workers within this system, both professional and non-professional.

Let me repeat: if nurses are to have any major impact on changing the law and on changing the economic structures in the world of work, our class struggles within nursing must be eliminated. The lack of unity we hear so much about in nursing is really an outgrowth of the phenomenon of classes constantly struggling and fighting. We must understand these struggles and these fights more fully. Knowing about the detrimental purposes they serve can help all of us overcome the conflicts we have about them. Knowledge alone can help nurses overcome the brainwashing we have been subjected to by the legal and economic systems paying us poorly and treating us poorly in exchange for our labor.

CONTROLLING NURSING'S PRODUCTION: NEW MODES FOR DELIVERING NURSING CARE

With nurses of all levels locked into the lowest paid positions in the health field, nurses will never obtain the means of controlling nursing's production. Legal and illegal strikes bring nurses very few gains when it comes to controlling their practice. Moreover, when nurses do strike they risk job-loss, starvation, sickness, and ruin. In view of the misery accompanying strikes, nurses must begin to look for alternatives, alternative actions more likely to result in achieving the ends we want. Also, the hassles surrounding legal collective bargaining are rarely equal to the worth of the meager gains growing out of the struggles and disputes involved in bargaining.

While working for changes in the law, nurses must consider taking the action of moving their practice out of present economic structures in control of delivering nursing care. This will mean the creation of new institutions and new modes of practice within nursing. Nurses are, to some extent, already experimenting with new forms of practice, but this experimentation must take place on a much broader scale than seen currently. Nurses, for example, are engaged in group practice, private practice, partnerships, and some have formed private professional corporations. Hopefully, going beyond these forms of practice, we will, in the future, see nurses owning and controlling nursing homes, and establishing nursing centers in communities, centers designed solely for the production of nursing care for citizens who need and want it.

At the beginning of this paper, I commented upon the need for an international movement, a movement concerning itself solely with the question of women's health. The efforts of nurses to create new modes of nursing practice and new institutions for the production of nursing care should be an integral part of the type of movement I have in mind. Women themselves have already started their own health movement and nurses could be of great help in strengthening this movement. With large numbers of women working with the nursing profession to bring about change, a new system of health care can become a reality, a system quite unlike the capitalistic system we have now which only seeks to profit off of disease. The prime focus of any new systems created must be human nourishment and human health approached from a wholistic viewpoint.

Having made this grand proposal about our severing the binding ties we have with a system that, in many instances, prevents nurses from practicing nursing, I want to stress again that oppressive laws restrict human behavior. They give rise to the stifling of persons and their self-image. A stifled self-image leads to suffering, to wasted talents, and to a lack of human growth.

Oppressive laws must go, freeing individuals to fully become what they can become within the realm of human potential. The laws of health are not compatible with oppressive laws as set forth by a discriminatory legal system. Florence Nightingale talked about the laws of health and the laws of nursing being one and the same. Nurses need the freedom, and must be given the opportunity, to discover just what the laws of health and the laws of nursing really are. We can only make these discoveries through our practice and through our research serving well the peoples who need a wholistic kind of human nourishment.

This voyage of discovery can, and should, become a festival of life and learning. Engaging in our own search and helping people in their search for healthy states of being should be a joyous adventure. As nurses, we cannot engage in this search until we have eliminated harassment from our own lives and work settings. This is the century for nursing's rebirth and renewal; this rebirth and renewal must begin with the self of each individual nurse. In each of us, we need to give birth to a new consciousness of who we are as persons. As we begin to care more and more for ourselves, our activities in the world of work and living will reflect healthy changes as well. We can change our laws. And, we can, with spirits renewed, force society to respect our professional rights, privileges, and freedom.

REFERENCES

1. Arendt, H. (1959). *The human condition* (p. 170). New York: Doubleday & Company, Inc., Anchor books edition.
2. Letter from Helen Archer to Jo Ann Ashley, December 8, 1976.
3. "Sick Pay Struggle Goes On," *Chart*, Vol. 73, No. 10 (December, 1976), p. 3. Official Publication of the Illinois Nurses' Association.
4. Galbraith, J. K. (1973). *Economics and the public purpose* (pp. 30, 31). New York: The New American Library, Inc.
5. *Ibid.*, p. 33.
6. *Ibid.*, pp. 32, 33.
7. Sheehy, G. (1976). *Passages: Predictable crises of adult life* (p. 199). New York: E. P. Dutton & Co., Inc.
8. Williams, W. A. (1964). *The great evasion* (pp. 19, 20). Chicago: Quadrangle Books.
9. Marx, K., & Engels, F. (1964, 1974). *The communist manifesto* (pp. 57, 58). New York: Simon & Schuster, Inc. and Washington Square Press.

Chapter 8

MOBILIZATION OF NURSING ENERGIES FOR CONSTRUCTIVE ACTION ON NATIONAL AND LOCAL LEVELS*

PREFACE

I am quite pleased to be invited to Milwaukee to have some dialogue with nurses concerned about debating or discussing our nursing situation and constructive action we can take to bring about improvements. Since the title of my paper is the "Mobilization of Nursing Energies for Constructive Action on National and Local Levels," I want to say at the outset that having such dialogue is the most constructive use to which we can put our energies. As nurses, we need to talk with each other openly and clearly; we need to reason together and come to an understanding of who we are and of where we want to go in the future. The future development of our profession depends upon us and our actions and the most intelligent thing we can do is to talk to each other and come to some consensus on directions for nursing in American society.

---

* Presented at the first Annual Dialogue With The Leaders sponsored by Columbia Hospital, Nursing Staff Development, University of Wisconsin-Milwaukee, September 11, 1975.

I know that you are probably more concerned about local considerations of what you can do in your work setting or in your district. Thus, I hope that in our dialogue all will feel free to discuss specific examples of difficulties you are having at the present. I want to stress this point because my paper is rather general in its viewpoint and focus. I have outlined broadly general areas where we need to concentrate our attention and energies on both national and local levels. However, the only way we can make the content presented meaningful to each of us is to discuss what our present concerns are about nursing practice.

To get our dialogue off the ground, I have outlined my thoughts in the following manner: I will comment upon our crisis in health care and its relationship to nursing; secondly, I will discuss patterns of behavior on the part of nurses from a historical point of view. Then, I will move into a discussion of mobilizing nursing energies for action. Finally, I will talk about the goal of constructive action and the need for affirmative action programs for upgrading nursing within hospital settings.

CRISIS IN HEALTH CARE

Within recent years the American health care system has been attacked by critics ranging from presidents of the United States to middle class and poor citizens all complaining that the system is a failure. The charge is repeatedly made that the nursing, medical, and health care needs of the people are not being met. Many claim that the poor and not-so-poor daily go without needed nursing and medical attention. As nurses, we know this is so.

Crisis intervention is now being proposed for the American health care system. The system is thought to be sick. In an historical examination of this system, one can easily conclude that the diagnosis is social pathology. Etiology of the disorder is sexual discrimination of a chronic nature, with symptoms of the condition apparent for well over a century. Here, I am of course, making reference to the longstanding existence of prejudice and sexual bias directed toward our profession of nursing.

Social systems built on irrational bias and prejudiced beliefs can only perpetuate underlying disorder, reflect chaos, and remain relatively ineffective. Leading men in the health field have persistently argued that the less educated nurses are, the better able they [nurses] become to provide health care. This is an historical argument that nurses have had to live with. Since nurses deliver most of the care to the sick, the suffering, and to those coping with social problems impinging upon their health, this argument has served as a convenient rationalization for keeping women in a subordinate position to men within the health care system.

Over the years, the vast majority of nurses have been convinced that we were intellectually inferior and less capable than men as authorities on matters of sickness and health. In reality, though no fault of our own, many of us have ended up being less capable and thus, provide examples of the inferiority expected to us. As a result, we as a society have had repeated crises within our health care system.

Society has really been the victim as a result of the lack of development of nurses. As nurses, we daily attempt to alleviate social ills related to disease and health and the better prepared we are to do so, the better the care we can make available to the public and our patients.

From my observations and from what nurses are telling me, the attitudes of medical men and hospital executives toward nurses give little promise of changing rapidly on the national scene. Current practices and expressed beliefs do not provide hopeful evidence even remotely indicative of sincere interest in real change. Repressive politics is one of our most pressing and serious problems in the hospital field.

Societal views of nurses also remain narrow, based on myths and misconceptions. The public is largely ignorant of the vital role of nursing in the health field. Therefore, change, if it is to come in the form of social and economic reforms, must be initiated by us nurses. Our mobilization of nursing energy and its constructive use is perhaps more important now than it has ever been.

Self-Defeating Behavior: Its Elimination

Before examining the use of nursing energies in stirring up social ferment for starting a movement to change attitudes, practices, and ultimately delivery systems in general, we need to look carefully at past behaviors on the part of individual nurses and on the part of organized nursing, behaviors which have been largely self-defeating. If we are to effectively mobilize our energies on national and local levels, we need to try to change some of these self-defeating behaviors so characteristic of us.

To illustrate our problems in this area more fully and to give some perspective on them, I want to share some historical insights with you. In the early years of nursing's development, leaders feared failure and were afraid that they would not succeed in their efforts to bring about social reforms in nursing education, practice, and in health care. Because of their fear and intimidation as women, our leaders decided to approach their problems by assuming a "conciliatory" attitude so as not to antagonize anyone (i.e., other nurses or dominant men in the health field).

In a very real sense, this was a grave mistake for our early leaders to make. But ever since the first decade of the century, this attitude has characterized the approach used by individual nurses and by organized nursing. Conforming to rules set by other groups, we have not been bold or aggressive, either privately in one-to-one relationships and certainly not publicly.

The delivery of health care in this country has always been a political matter. People, of course, be they men or women, using a timid approach or stance do not survive in the world of politics. Groups using a timid approach cannot become socially visible and effective in a democracy, not in local communities or on state and national levels. In a democracy, people do inevitably have opposing viewpoints and disagreements are a part of life, the most real part for that matter. Disagreement and conflict are a part of healthy growth and development. People must fight for their ideas and beliefs openly and publicly in a nation where people reason together and come to some conclusion on what is best for individuals and the public welfare.

To always have an attitude of conforming to someone else's views, being conciliatory or non-antagonizing all the time is very detrimental to growth and psychological vitality on the part of a profession or an individual. But this has been the pattern in nursing, a pattern established long ago because nurses were women living in a world dominated by men. Historically, nurses were afraid to actively express their viewpoints openly, and this is still a reality because we are still predominantly women and still hesitant to publicly express what we believe in, and feel, and think about certain issues.

We need to use our energies differently in the future. As we become more politically outspoken and hopefully visible to the public, we must remember there is a time for *compromise,* a time to *concede,* a time to be *agreeable,* but that time *is not* when the battle is on and we are fighting for a cause or attempting to have our ideas accepted by others. The fight in life, when one lives in a democracy such as ours, is an intellectual one, and a continuous one at that.

Only those who persist can win for their side or for their cause. Those who behave in an appeasing manner from the beginning lose out, get lost in the shuffle, and ultimately waste their energies in the process of attempting to influence decisions vital to them and vital to society. We nurses frequently lose a great deal by our tendencies to avoid controversy and conflict. Conflict and fighting for one's rights and beliefs promote growth. To avoid these or to deny the need for confrontation is to settle for stagnation, or it is to die slowly from one ailment or another. At least, to deny the need for confrontation is to deny the need for growth and progress.

That nurses lack persistence and avoid heated exchanges of ideas and viewpoints is just as evident within local practice settings as it is on the political and social fronts at the national and state levels. All too frequently, nurses willingly agree with other professionals about given decisions regarding health care; also, we as a profession quite frequently have no impact on bringing about change or in having our ideas accepted where improving nursing care is the issue.

Historically, our profession failed to have any great impact on health care policies and delivery system because nurses were not the shapers or makers of decisions and policies. On the part of early and some current leaders in nursing, conciliatory attitudes assumed to avoid failure have been and are really coping mechanisms, and cope we nurses have for years. Men in the health field have used this attitude against us time and time again to foster their own causes.

These attitudes have not, moreover, served to create unity in the profession but divisiveness. Conciliatory and noncommittal behavior has led and leads to persisting antagonism and conflict among various groups within nursing, notably between educators and practitioners, or between practitioners and nursing administrators.

I must stress here that I am not advocating conformity or uniformity of viewpoints on the part of nurses, but clearness in communication with the public and with each other about nursing's role and our contributions to health care. In our dialogue tonight we can discuss specific methods and practical approaches we can begin to use in working on changing our attitudes and our behavior patterns in order to move away from the use of energies in a self-defeating manner.

Mobilizing Nursing Energies for Constructive Action

I would like for us to turn our attention to ways in which we as a profession can use our energies to increase our social visibility, on national and local levels. First, I want to comment on nursing's relation to health care policies. We have not had a major impact in this area and this is one reason we are constantly confronted with the charge that our health care system is lacking in quality. We cannot have quality care without creating a greater public emphasis on the importance of nursing care, which is the heart and core of health care. We live in a society that grossly devalues both nurses and nursing care. This is a situation we must change for the sake of ourselves and American citizens.

Organized nursing (by which I mean the A.N.A. as well as state and local districts) needs to formulate definite and specific policies reflecting vision and perceptiveness regarding the nursing needs of society and the ways and means by which nurses can better accomplish their social mission in seeing that these needs are more adequately met. Public pressure originating at the local level must be directed toward formulating national health policies which will insure the full utilization of women's abilities and talents.

For nurses, patients, and society in general, time has been wasted because organized nursing has been slow, slow in formulating policies and public statements urging more rapid and constructive changes in the health field. Our's has not been a public voice that has been heard. Defeatist behavior of collaborating and cooperating in the support of policies and practices undermining nursing's progress will have to be replaced with new and different approaches.

Political developments on both national and local levels warrant careful examination. Intelligent decisions have to be made in regard to their relevance to nursing and health care delivery. Political pressures within the health field are and will continue to be largely financial in nature on both national and local levels. The lack of financial support for nursing has constituted a major impediment to our development in the past. Political astuteness and activism are essential for insuring that this does not occur in the future.

Political pressure is also necessary in the area of gaining an appropriate legal status for nurses, a status that recognizes us as a profession separate and apart from one needing medical supervision. The legal system has served as a major oppressive force for nursing by perpetuating the myth of medical supervision. In the vast majority of states this condition still exists. Policies regarding the legal protection of both nurses and the public are essential as a means of ultimately insuring the freedom of nurses to provide professional care in practice settings. Largely because nurses have had a second-class legal status and few rights and privileges as professionals practice has been, in many instances, narrow in scope and limited in its potential.

Professional inequality is a major problem for nursing to deal with today. Equal rights and privileges can only be obtained by influencing the legislative process. This will involve changing public opinion and gaining general support for nursing policies. Public exposure of discriminatory practices directed toward nurses is an important activity that should begin to receive the greater part of our attention and energies. The public is largely unaware of discriminatory practices directed toward nurses. Providing correct information to the public about employment practices and the conditions in which we work will be a necessary step in changing traditional treatment and attitudes toward us.

Another problem requiring the attention of political activists is the control which organized medicine exerts over our profession. The efforts of medicine to control nursing never cease. Definite action to alter this type of behavior is indicated. Medical men appoint themselves as public spokesmen for nursing. As a result of their lack of information on and, respect for nursing, the public is often misinformed and nursing's image is damaged. Both national, state, and local groups in nursing should demand the disbandment of all medical committees on nursing. Public statements about the harmful effects of such committees need to be formulated and presented to various groups interested in health care, especially those instrumental in making policies.

Only nurses know enough about our field to formulate public statements about nursing. Should medical groups need information about nursing, they can communicate directly with nursing groups. If joint decisions need to be made, nursing and medicine can equally join together for the purpose of mutually deciding upon the stand each shall take regarding an issue of importance to both, and the public should know of the reasoning of both groups.

Historically, medical committees on nursing have always served a political function. Their reports are usually dispensed widely to physicians as well as to other groups such as politicians, hospital officials, and the public. As public spokesmen for nursing, medical men perpetuate their own biased views about what is best for nursing. This paternalistic attitude helps no one; it does not help the public and it certainly does not help nurses.

On the national scene and in local hospital settings, physicians have, in the past, had control over information and communication about nursing. Their views and decisions are often not based on fact. Permitting medicine to maintain this type of control over information and therefore, decision-making about nursing, will be detrimental to nursing from a political, economic, and professional standpoint. And, because of the power and influence of medicine, public support for nursing policies will be more difficult to achieve.

In the event that medical groups do not disband their special interest committees, organized nursing as a part of its political strategy should form its own committees on medicine at the district, state, and national levels. The purpose of these committees should not be that of making decisions about medical practice or education. Instead, nursing committees on medicine should serve as a countervailing force to offset, to impede, and to eliminate in the public mind the validity and reliability of medical reports and opinions on nursing.

Other functions of these committees could include collecting information on what medicine is saying about nursing, who receives this information, what do the latter think of it and plan to do with it. After careful examination of the accuracy, intent, and purpose of medical declarations on nursing matters, the next step is to publicly clarify, and if discriminatory, disqualify what is being said and publicized. Also, nursing's own position on a given issue can be set forth for the public to examine and compare with those formulated by groups involved in the health care system.

Both public and private confrontations with domineering physicians and hospital administrators are inevitable in the future. Although open confrontation will probably be unpleasant for most of us nurses, revealing underlying truth, having open and honest discussion, and feeling free to express one's own thoughts, will ultimately be of service to the public, to nurses, and to the health care system by improving the quality of care we can provide. As nurses, we need to give our undivided attention and wholehearted support to nursing. Devoting our loyalties to other groups is self-defeating behavior.

PROFESSIONAL EQUALITY FOR NURSES: THE GOAL OF CONSTRUCTIVE ACTION

Achieving more equitable and fair treatment of nursing practitioners in health care delivery systems will require the use of strategies involving political, economic, and psychological factors, with the latter especially important for changing attitudes and behavior patterns. Better working conditions with the built in provisions of fair economic rewards for responsibility assumed and attractive professional incentives will not be easy to accomplish.

The value of professional nursing care is often minimized for economic reasons alone. This is blatant discrimination against us and against our profession. This discrimination needs our most careful scrutiny. In no other profession or occupation are the more highly educated and skilled discriminated against as they are in nursing. The public does not know that this type of discrimination is almost universally present in health care settings. The public is often deceived into thinking it is getting the best nursing care possible when, in reality, this is far from the truth.

It would be of value to organize a campaign, both locally and nationally, for the purpose of educating the public on this particular issue. The public is exploited as much as nurses by this type of discrimination. Encouraging public questioning of the qualifications of all health professionals is especially important at this time with the current proliferation of physician assistant's and other health workers with varying kinds of preparation. The public, unless they ask and are told, cannot know who is competent to give care and who is not.

To become equal participants in policy and decision-making processes which affect nursing, all nurses need their self-confidence increased. Aggressive confrontation and the development of other strategies cannot come from those who are inhibited by oppression and unaware of the effects of this oppression on their lives and professional growth and development.

Long-standing social discrimination has curious effects on individuals. We nurses may need to be repeatedly reminded that we are an oppressed group and that we are human and not anonymous stereotyped creatures whose sole responsibility is to the sick. We owe something to ourselves before we can ever fully direct our energies to the betterment of society. If we nurses are to climb out of our oppression and create a better future for practitioners in our field, we will need to learn the skills necessary for the move from subjection to freedom. Such a move will entail conflict and controversy. However, as indicated earlier, conflicts (both internal and external) are a part of the process of growth itself.

Group awareness, cohesiveness, and an organized movement to accomplish change will be forthcoming when we nurses collectively identify with the cause of women's rights and equal justice where developing our potential is concerned. Society needs what we have to offer. Identification with and knowledge of feminist strategies and tactics can be of tremendous educational value to us nurses. Many problems confronting us nurses are somewhat unique because of our role and responsibility in the care of the sick. Nonetheless, there are few actions which could be taken that would cause more abuses in patient care than those existing already in our American health care system.

AFFIRMATIVE ACTION PROGRAMS FOR WOMEN IN HEALTHCARE SETTINGS

As nurses and as a profession, we are confronted with the basic problem of social injustice and inequality. Historically, both local hospitals, organized medicine and organized hospital administration, and the whole of society have directed prejudice toward us. The social consequences of this prejudice should receive our utmost attention. By mobilizing our energies we can hope to correct some of the defects and confusion so obvious within our American health care system and within nursing.

Social justice cannot be obtained without specific actions and strategies. Programs and activities for achieving social justice should be the focus of local and national efforts. Within recent years, we have heard a lot about affirmative action programs within universities and within other economic and social institutions. Institutions are now required by law to plan programs that will upgrade the status of women and other minorities, especially their economic status and recognition of abilities. These programs are designed to eliminate discrimination and to foster equal treatment of men and women, where gross inequality is evident.

If we, as a profession, are to bring about favorable change, we cannot avoid capitalizing on this significant societal development. In addition to collective bargaining, nurses need to insist upon having positive and definite programs of affirmative action to aid nurses in upgrading their status and opportunities for advancement in both the professional and economic world. Right now, with repressive politics operative at a peak, we need affirmative action officers within our hospital settings, just as we have them in universities. Every district within organized nursing the nation over needs to explore the ramifications of affirmative action for nurses within districts and states.

Affirmative action officers could be responsible for the careful evaluation of hiring and firing policies within hospitals, promotions and pay increases for nurses and for the elimination of discriminatory practices inherent in no differential pay for our more highly educated within nursing. Recruitment efforts should also be included within the range of responsibility of such a person. For example, to what extent do hospitals seek out and employ our most highly prepared in the field of nursing to staff hospitals. With the aid of someone informed of the latest legal and social guidelines set up by the Equal Employment Opportunity Commission, all kinds of grievances and concerns of nurses could be challenged and appealed. If we are to use our energies constructively, we need to take this opportunity to use every legal and social means available to have our professional expertise recognized and adequately paid for by our employers.

We now have N-CAP at the national level and on many state levels to help us be informed and visible in the political arena. Collective bargaining efforts are also underway. But, in local settings, we need more affirmative action than these to insure the upgrading of our status, and to insure progress. Public pressure and specific legal pressures will be essential to bring about the achievement of professional equality for us nurses.

We are dealing with a system that has a long history of oppressing nurses and this system will yield to nothing but force, since nursing (for a century) has been viewed as of peripheral importance where the economic operation of hospitals is concerned. It is this view of nursing which we must change. We want equality of treatment and its accompanying responsibilities. We want opportunities and the means of realizing our potential as professional members of society who have a great deal to offer in improving health care. Professional nursing means quality care. And, it is time we ended the exploitation of the public and began to provide American citizens with a bit of quality care for a change.

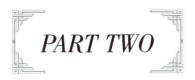

PART TWO

FEMINISM AND NURSING

Women have by no means monopolized the nursing field since monks, knights, mendicant friars, and many other groups of men have shared the toil in earlier days. It is perfectly plain however that many of the difficulties which nurses faced in the past were due to the social, educational, and economic hardships that affected women particularly. All of these have not disappeared entirely, but they are much less formidable than they used to be, thanks to feminists and others who brought the struggle out into the open and cleared away at least a few of the old impediments.

Dock and Stewart, 1938, p. 367

*T*hroughout its history, nursing has experienced a curious relationship with feminism. Viewed as women's work for most of this century, nursing has been both embraced and disdained by feminists. The contradictory nature of nursing work poses a conundrum for feminists. On the one hand, nursing is appealing because of the value placed on caring and compassion, yet on the other hand, it is disdained as subordinate to medicine. Similarly, feminism has been a source of tension and contradiction to nursing. During feminism's second wave in the 1970s, nurses struggled with their relation to the women's movement. Often ignored or criticized by feminist groups such as NOW, nurse feminists began uniting to forge a feminist perspective on nursing. Consciousness raising groups emerged and, over time, nursing saw the emergence of feminist groups such as Nurse

Now, Democratic-socialist nurse (DSA-nurses), and Cassandra. The words of Jo Ann Ashley cracked opened the consciousness of numerous nurses in this era. She admonished nurses not to turn their backs on feminism once again. She hoped that, by coming to terms with their history as women, nurses would be able to end their typically oppressed group behaviors and unify. Dr. Ashley embraced feminism as a theoretical perspective that could guide social activism to better the lives of women.

As the women's movement evolved in the 1970s, three distinct perspectives emerged: liberal feminism, socialist feminism, and radical feminism (Fee, 1975). While Dr. Ashley began her writing from the standpoint of liberal feminism, over time her writing became more influenced by socialist and radical feminism. From the standpoint of liberal feminism, Dr. Ashley argued for equality in education and the workplace and political opportunities. Her early writings on power and politics suggest that she believed that equality was attainable within the established systems of politics, education, and employment. As her perspectives matured, however, her writings also reflected an integration of socialist and radical feminist perspectives. The concepts "patriarchy" and "oppression" drew her to the work of contemporary feminists such as Mary Daly, Barbara Ehrenreich, Adrian Rich, and Rosemary Ruether. The result was the legitimation of feminism to nursing and the valuing of nursing by feminists and scholars in the field of women's studies.

The two papers in this section present Dr. Ashley's thought on the relationship between nursing and feminism. The first paper, written in the early 1970s and published in the *American Journal of Nursing* in 1975, was intended to raise the consciousness of nurses to the historic relationship of nursing to feminism. Writing from a liberal feminist perspective, Ashley criticizes nurses for their anti-feminism. Citing nursing leader and feminist Lavinia Dock as a rare exception, Ashley reiterates Dock's warning, writing "that if nurses are to attain equality as professionals in the health field they must challenge the male dominance . . . only by understanding nursing history can nurses break the oppressive chains of the past." Ashley and Dock are united in nursing history as risk taking feminist nurses and historians.

The second paper, "Power in Structured Misogyny: Implications for the Politics of Care," was published by *Advances in Nursing Science* in 1980. Peggy L. Chinn, then ANS Editor, as a friend and colleague of Dr. Ashley, encouraged her to write such "interpretative political analyses." As the lead paper in this collection, it describes the role of misogyny or "hatred of women" in shaping the politics of care. Framed as a radical feminist analysis of nursing, the paper shows how misogynist ideas have found support as much in religious ideas as in social institutions and traditions. Ashley suggests that nursing has been shaped by misogynist ideas of women which then serve as effective means of social control. Stereotyped as angels of mercy, and demeaned as inferior to medicine, nurses have been mired in a culture of ambivalence. Noddings (1989) elaborates that this stereotypical view of women as good and evil has led to viewing women as " 'angel[s] in the house.' Women have been credited with natural goodness, an innate allegiance to 'a law of kindness.' But this same description extols her as infantile, weak, and mindless—a creature in constant need of male supervision and protection" (p. 59).

Dr. Ashley suggests that long-standing social conceptions of women as evil, inferior, and subordinate are inherent in the foundations of many theories from Maslow to Freud. She describes the power of patriarchy to perpetuate social equalities through social structure and ideology. From her analysis, Ashley also proposes this imperative: to unmask misogynist ideology in theories and bodies of knowledge as actual threats to the health and the potential of nursing. She cautions that in the pursuit of professional status many nurses have joined with patriarchal forces to perpetuate the "token torture" of other women. Ashley's impassioned plea for nurses to make meaningful connection with other nurses and other women to establish a community of caring should not go unnoticed even today. Ashley states "I believe nursing cannot become self-directing or effective in the politics of care without embracing feminism and all that it stands for."

Ashley also urges nurses to draw on feminism as an energy source for theory building. She embraces the power of language as fundamental to ending the hold of patriarchy. According to Ashley, feminism could provide the theoretical basis for nursing to effectively study phenomena that threaten the health of women. This viewpoint stood in stark contrast to the trend in nursing, then more than now, but still significant even now, to emulate the positivist approach of "objective science." Ashley took the stance, drawn from feminist and women's studies, that research should begin to study the *experiences* of women including nurses. To the credit of ANS, this paper stands as one of the few publications on the theoretical consideration of feminism for nursing. Dr. Ashley introduced a generation of nurses to the critique of patriarchy and to the potential of feminism. Her writings helped to build a bridge between the disciplines of nursing and women's studies.

References

1. Dock, L., & Stewart, I. M. (1938). *A short history of nursing.* New York: G. P. Putnum.
2. Fee, E. (1975). Women and health care: A comparison of theories. *International Journal of Health Services, 5*(3).
3. Noddings, N. (1989). *Women and evil.* Berkeley: University of California Press.

Upside Down and Inside Out

by Jo Ann Ashley

What face do I show the world,
And why?
Do I feel that the world will
Not like me with my upside
Down and my inside out?
I hardly like myself the way
I am now.
Why does the world give me
Trouble too?

Would I really be happier inside
If I turned my upside down and
My inside out?
My soul urges me to do so.
I need to grow.
Some people love my upside.
They tell me so, and praise me
As I come and go.
I have helped them in some way,
I know.

It is all very, very good to be
Liked so,
But would these same people like
Me
If my upside were down and my
Inside out.
I must let these praising people
Know that they do oppress my spirit
So.
My greatest urge and need right now
Is to put my upside down and my inside
Out,
But I do fear I will not be liked for
What I am inside.

I am scared of what is inside too.
I have sought to please for all of
My life.
I am good.
I am kind.
I am a woman.
I am a nurse.

I have never been anything but these,
Good, kind, pleasing.
My inside, if it were up, would hate
All of these in me.

I would like to put my inside out
For this is really me.
That side is surely also good and
Kind,
But it will not try so hard to please.
It will just seek to be free, alive,
Well, and healthy.

My upside I have lived with, my
Upside I have known.
My inside is a stranger to me.
In order to free my soul, and live
And breathe I am going to put my
Upside down and bring my inside
Out.

My upside is false.
My inside is real.
To put the false down, to let the
Real out is what I seek.
This I will do though it will hurt
And disappoint a few.
But as things stand now I am hurting
Me
By keeping my upside out and my inside
Down.
I need to reverse these.

Someday I will curse the social order
That has forced me to live with my
Upside out and my inside down.
I have not been free.
My only task now is to change this
Order in me.
By doing this I will set a part of
Society free,
The part that exists in me.

Chapter 9

NURSING AND EARLY FEMINISM*

At the turn of the century, women did not have any political status, not even the right to vote. They were not legally or socially free even to take part in public debates on their welfare. Early fighters were determined and did persist in efforts to obtain the vote. They were less persistent in other vital matters, however, and thus equal rights for women is still the most pressing political issue confronting women. Obtaining the right to vote was only a minute step toward equal rights.

As in the past, women are relatively powerless today and politically and economically dependent on the decisions of men. This reality operates very often both at home and at work for married, divorced, or single women. The historical failure of women to achieve independence grew out of lack of persistence in changing the oppressive social order.

A contemporary critic of the early feminist movement has classified the women of the day into two groups, radicals and conservatives.[1] The outspoken radicals were the ones who went to jail and endured "embarrassment, mobbings, beatings, even hunger strikes" to win the vote. The views of these feminists were characterized by a concern for the total growth of women as human beings, participating equally with men in society. This same critic argues that the conservatives

---

*Reprinted with permission from *American Journal of Nursing* (1975).

were antifeminists. They did not show serious concern about the social and political problems faced by women in society. They did not act to ensure the achievement of their rights to develop and to function independently of men in professions or society.

Efforts of radicals resulted in obtaining the vote, but because of the larger influence of conservatives, women obtained little else. After suffrage became a reality, most women went about their daily work and forgot all about the fight for real freedom. They ended up devoting attention to causes having little or nothing to do with the elevation of their oppression as a class. Instead, they provided visible and invisible support for a political and social order that denied them the rights and privileges accorded to men. Thus both radicals and conservatives failed of major changes in societal values and institutions.

Historically, it is highly significant that professional women were among the conservatives, with nurses no exception. Professional women joined all the "good causes," causes good not for them but for the male-dominated institutions that represented them. These women assumed very narrow political and social positions, devoting attention not to changing the social order itself, but to limited problems related to their own educational and professional development, whatever their occupation. Thus, women have remained an oppressed class, having made little progress in the professional world which men still dominate.

Nurses as Anti-Feminists

To the detriment of their own growth as professional persons, nurses were among the most conservative of the conservatives. With rare exception, they were nonfeminists. Early leaders overlooked their second-class status as women and identified with limited movement, such as the development of hospitals as businesses.

The failure of nurses to identify with radical feminists seeking to change the social order led to the failure of the nursing profession to liberate both education and practice. Nurse education was absorbed into hospital management and the economic value and use of women in hospitals was a major factor enabling politically astute groups to grow and prosper at the expense of nurses. Nurses were not the equals of physicians in the political and economic spheres, and so nursing's continuing subjection to male dominance resulted. Other than providing efficient care for the sick, nurses have had little influence on hospital development in this country, though they did much to reform hospital care in the nineteenth century. But with nursing support, hospitals developed as big business—with further oppression of women in the health field.

Nurses and Male Dominance

Male dominance is a problem for women in the whole of society, but nurses have special problems in this respect. Organized hospital administration and physicians opposed any reforms by nurses. Many early administrators were medical men, and physicians did not want nurses to organize. They objected to the claim of nurses that they could have professional status equal to that of physicians. Before and after 1910, physicians heatedly argued that nursing had overstepped its bounds, going too far in erecting nursing as a profession "controlled by women nurses."[2]

Most nursing leaders of the time did not seriously question male dominance in the health field, nor did they question the serious and long-range effects of women's subjugation to men. Lavinia L. Dock was a rare exception. As a radical feminist, Ms. Dock warned her colleagues that the threat of male dominance was the major problem confronting the nursing profession. In 1903, Ms. Dock spoke with some insight on developments that were destined to ensure male dominance:

A quest-determined movement on the part of certain elements of our masculine brothers to seize and guide the helm of the new teaching is...most undeniably in progress. Several of these same brothers have lately openly asserted themselves in printed articles as the founders and leaders of that nursing education, which, so far as it has gone, we all know to have been worked out by the brains, bodies, and souls of the women to whom this paper is addressed, and who have often had to win their points in clinched opposition to the will of these same brothers, and solely by dint of their own personal prestige as women.[3]

Ms. Dock urged leaders to think in terms of their "latent" and "unsuspected power" and the ways it could be used to overcome threats of male dominance. Resentful of professional injustices and indignities suffered by nurses in their contacts with "overbearing" medical men and hospital administrators, she reminded nurses that those who engaged in the continuing abuse of women were neither friends nor benefactors of nursing or women. She emphasized that organized nursing was ineffective as a force speaking out on public questions of concern to women.

The movement toward male dominance which Ms. Dock identified was successful. Nursing leaders ignored all her warnings and in the second decade of the century actually became non-voting members of the American Hospital Association.[4] They worked with physicians and administrators on joint committees, expecting their oppressors to help them solve nursing problems. They sought approval from men, not liberation. As a result, from the first decade of the century onward, physicians and hospital administrators have remained in positions of dominance and control over nursing and health care.

Becoming accomplices to their own subordination is not unique to nurses. Women in general usually comply with systems that keep them oppressed. This behavior on the part of nursing leaders was, however, especially damaging to the efforts of their own professional organizations and to improving the status of nurses. Male-dominated professions made rapid progress, but the advance of nursing is slowed to this day. By identifying narrowly with hospital development, nurses did, in fact, help maintain male dominance. Their position as conservatives cooperating with men prevented their bringing about reforms in the social order that might have elevated the status of all women, since nursing is the largest female profession in society.

Second-class citizenship brought second-class professionalism as well. The apprenticeship system of education subjected nurses to the male authority of hospital administrators. Moreover, early nurse practice acts did not provide professional privileges or protection for nurses, only restriction of their independent actions. Already bound to an inferior educational system and male authority, nurses obtained only the right to practice nursing under the supervision of physicians, not the recognition that they were the professional equals of physicians with rights to practice independently.

The legal subjection of nurses to physicians has persisted into the present decade, with only a few states having enacted new laws that recognize nurses as independent practitioners. Nurse practice acts supported the myth of female dependency and their need for male supervision, and in so doing have perpetuated the myth of medical supervision. With the exception of carrying out doctors' orders, nurses have seldom or never actually been supervised by physicians. Medical supervision is not and never has been a reality in many practice settings.

Another quotation from Lavinia Dock best describes why the nursing profession has not openly confronted male dominance and sexual discrimination. Nursing, she said in 1903, "has not made itself a moral force, is not a public conscience, takes not position in large public questions: is not feared by those of low standards, allows all manner of new conditions and developments in nursing affairs to arise, flourish, succeed, or fail."[5]

Instead of openly questioning sexual prejudice directed toward nurses, leaders, without public protest, accepted it and lived silently with the results. With paternalism legalized and apprenticeship institutionalized in nursing, the oppression of nurses was built into the laws of the land and into the educational system. The end result has been that of the continuing low social status of nurses and gross economic discrimination in the woman's profession. As commonly observed in fields of women's work, nursing has been associated more with labor and domestic services than it has been with professions having prestige. Low pay and few economic rewards for the average nurses (and even our best educated) remain realities, even though in many parts of the country organized nursing's economic security efforts have brought about significant improvement.

Actually one need not go back as far in time as Lavinia Dock for evidence of nurses docility under male dominance. Shirley Titus, speaking on the economic security program (in which she had been a prime mover) at the 1952 ANA convention, spoke of "nursing's long social slumber" and pointed out that at a time when other workers had succeeded in markedly reducing their work week, nurses were still working a 48 hour week or even longer. She remarked, "Both organized medicine and the hospital have always sought to assume active and positive direction of nursing affairs in order that both nurses and nursing should function in a way that would best serve their special interests. These controls have prevented nurses from security that background and experience which would have prepared them to live more fully and function more effectively in the present social scene.[6]

Legal restraints and economic abuses have prevented nurses from realizing their highest ambitions of becoming equals of men in professions. Career commitments have not been stressed in nursing. Both physicians and hospital administrators repeatedly argued that nurses could make their main contributions to society by becoming wives and mothers. The myth that women exist to be mothers has fostered male dominance in the health field as much as it has in society at large. This myth has been used as a means of urging nurses not to compete economically with men for monetary rewards in the health field.

Inequality in the health field is the major problem facing nurses today, as it is for women in general. Current research exploring the world of women's work shows that, in comparison to the progress of men, "women are falling behind," and that could lose nurses some of the gains their economic security program has brought them. Moreover, "women have not displaced or even seriously challenged male dominance."[7] If nurses are to prevent failure in the future, they must carefully evaluate their position of inequality in the social order and design public political action to bring about improvements. Only by understanding nursing's history can nurses break the oppressive chains of the past. The main lesson to learn from history is how not to repeat the events of the past. The main lesson to learn from history is how not to repeat the errors of the past. Today, identification with the feminist cause and obtaining equality with men in the health field is a must.

There seem to be brighter signs on the horizon. The American Nurses' Association has brought suit in nine cases of discrimination against women in university faculty pension plans. Nurses are joining the National Organization of Women in fair numbers. A nurse, Wilma Scott Heide, has served NOW as its very active president. And now there is Nurses NOW, with several chapters across the country working to advance the cause of women.[8] This time the movement may be successful.

REFERENCES

1. Firestone, S. (1971). *Dialectic of Sex, The Case for Feminist Revolution* (pp. 15–21). New York: Bantam Books.
2. Satterthwaite, T. E. (1910, January). Private nurses and nursing: With recommendation for their betterment. *New York Medical Journal*, 91.
3. Dock, L. L. The duty of this society in public work. In *Proceedings of the Tenth Annual Convention of the American Society of Superintendents of Training Schools*, held at Pittsburgh, October 7–8, 1904 (pp. 78–79).
4. *See* American Hospital Association. Transactions. Chicago: *The Association*, 1913, p.91.
5. Dock, *op.cit.* pp. 77–79.
6. Titus, S. C. (1952, September). Economic facts of life for nurses. *American Journal of Nursing*,(52), 1109–1112.
7. Epstein, C. E., & Goody, W. J. (Eds.). (1971). *Other Half Roads to Women's Equality* (p. 76). Englewood Cliffs, NJ: Prentice Hall.
8. Nurses form own NOW (N) *American Journal of Nursing*, (75), 200. Feb. 1975.

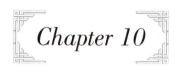

Chapter 10

POWER IN STRUCTURED MISOGYNY

Implications for the Politics of Care*

So while I do not pray for anybody or any party to
commit outrages
Still do *I pray*, and that earnestly and constantly
For some terrific shock
To startle the women of this nation into self respect
Which will compel them to see the abject degradation of
Their present position;
Which will make them proclaim their allegiance to women
First:
Which will enable them to see that man can no more feel,
Speak, or act for woman than could the old slave holder
For his slave.
The fact is, women are in chains.
And their servitude is all the more debasing because they
Do not realize it.
O, to compel them to see and feel.
And to give them the courage and conscience to speak and
Act for their own freedom.
Though they face the scorn and contempt of all the world
For doing it.

Susan B. Anthony, 1870

* Reprinted with permission of Aspen Publishers, Inc. © 1980. From *ANS/Politics of Care*, (1980), Vol. 2 (no. 3), pp. 3–22.

INTRODUCTION

The purpose of this article is to show how misogyny, or the hatred of women, has been historically structured throughout human experience and to interpret how this structured misogyny affects our current politics of care. In confronting destructive elements in patriarchy, nurses must intellectually and emotionally come to grips with the extent to which patriarchal ideas, institutions and practice weaken and destroy nursing's power, practice and ability to exercise effective politics in care. Coming to grips with the damaging effects of patriarchy is necessary before nurses can begin to visualize new ways of thinking, acting and being at home and at work.

Within patriarchy the power of structured misogyny keeps women in their role of glorified servants to men—keeps them oppressed in subjugated domestic roles living out the cult of true womanhood. Great women scholars and writers have for centuries recognized and analyzed this basic fact and its effect on the course of human history. The present generation of women scholars has built on this heritage and is now showing more clearly than ever how misogyny has been structured into patriarchal relations, philosophies, theories, myths, language and totality of human experience. They have shown how misogyny has contributed to the destructive course of history and why we now seem to be at the end of a patriarchal founded civilization.

Since the vast majority of nurses are women, our first concern must be that of analyzing the various forms of violence leading to the constant destruction of the mental and physical health of women. Remaining deaf, dumb and blind to the suffering and destruction of our own kind is agreeing to the political dominance of those who wish to continue destroying the strengths of women.

EARTHLY AND HUMAN DEVASTATION

We are living in a time period when the exhaustion of the earth's resources, when disregard for human and nonhuman life is rapidly leading to forms of earthly and human devastation, such as dehumanization by computerization and nuclear destruction, which are hard to imagine by the American mind. We live in a society that no longer values the capacity to care for human life. Our society values technology, machines and its structures of steel and concrete more than it values life itself.[1]

Humans are not made of steel. They are not made of cement or of concrete. They live. They breathe. They feel. Humans are not made of wood or of iron. They bleed when cut. They cry when badly hurt. They fear when fright takes hold of their hearts. The structure of the human body and mind is such that it requires nourishment to survive. Both body and mind require an atmosphere and environment conducive to the maintenance of life. We live in a society that negates this. Our society overlooks the nature of human beings and the nature of the earth on which we live.[1, 2]

Slowly but surely, writers and scholars are beginning to take note of the limits (i.e., the seeming inability of people in general to reverse the exploitation) surrounding the exploitation of the earth's resources and of human life. As one cultural historian puts it: "We have already entered the era of limits, and with industrial expansion at its limit, people are beginning to look at other things for the meaning of human culture . . ." This male historian notes that the 21st century "will see all the worst nightmares of the ecologists come true in epidemics of environmentally caused diseases which will recall the Black Death of medieval times."[1]

Feminist scholars are currently pinpointing the origins of the runaway course of earthly and human destruction observed in society.[1,2,3,4] Rosemary Ruether explains that "only today have large numbers of people begun to suspect that patriarchy, which has shaped human history until now, is unviable for future development and indeed is fast proving unable to maintain the survival of humankind on the planet.[2] In other words, patriarchal ideas have given shape and form to social institutions, lifestyles and governments that are now proving inadequate to preserve human life and the earth itself.

Death in Life

Although in most of our present life experiences it appears that the sources of patriarchal institutions remain powerful and strong, a close historical analysis reveals that our present civilization is crumbling. Most of recorded history reveals that men are and always have been dominant in this world.[2,3,5] As a result, our lifestyles and our social institutions are built on sand. The patriarchal foundations, which are grounded in marriage and the nuclear family, are not firm. Indeed the foundations are shaking. They are feeble, frail and falling. It is past the time for patriarchy to cease being dominant. Valuing patriarchy has meant death in life—malaise, apathy, depression, and general destruction of the human spirit—for many, and in the future it promises to mean death in life for many more. It is questionable whether the well-intentioned people of this earth can reverse the human political and environmental destruction that patriarchy has left behind.[3]

The death in life resulting from patriarchy has tremendous implications for the politics of care. Nursing will have to prepare itself to care for the victims of epidemics of environmentally caused diseases and the Black Death of the future.[1] The patriarchy has done little and is doing little to stop the evils causing these diseases and this death.[2,3,6]

As the recent Three Mile Island incident clearly demonstrates, our civilization faces widespread and possibly lethal outcomes from the uses of nuclear energy, and seems unable to come to grips with how to reverse or stop the events leading to destruction. As radical feminist Mary Daly clearly points out, the patriarchal leaders are unable or unwilling to stop their own destructive games.[3] Daly stresses the fact that our society is necrophilic, in love with death and unconcerned about life. Patriarchal scientists and leaders "through the 'peaceful use of nuclear energy' and other forms of pure pollution . . . have paved the way for planetary plagues causing disgusting and virulent sores—radiation sickness and various forms of cancer."[3] From a political and caring standpoint, nurses would be wise to actively and publicly oppose the forces giving rise to the ultimate destruction of human health on this earth.

ROOTS OF STRUCTURED MISOGYNY IN
RELIGION AND PHILOSOPHY

Misogyny and hatred of the expansion of women's potential beyond the male-defined limits of serving males find their greatest support in religious ideas, traditions and institutions. As Ruether explains, "The religion of patriarchal culture validates this auxiliary status of women in various ways . . . In the creation story, genetic humanity is envisioned as male, the essential and original autonomous human person. Woman was created second as a derivative being."[4] Myths surrounding the cult of true womanhood permeate patriarchal history. Because of myths accompanying pervasive misogyny, nurses are still the servants of physicians and secretaries the servants of business executives.

Women as Evil

In patriarchal religion, men alone were created in the image of god. Misogynous myths portray women as evil instead of being created in god's image. The biblical "misogynist tradition goes beyond the definitions of women in terms of property dependency and service. It defines women as the source of evil and, in some sense, inherently evil. This of course is suggested in the stories that make Eve not only secondary in creation but the source of sin in the world, either through the fall from Paradise or by the seduction of the angels through which the demonic beings were born."[4]

The association of women with evil is a predominant thought in all written history and mythology.[2,4] According to Simone de Beauvoir, "That is why religious and codes of law treat woman with such hostility as they do . . . Eve, given to Adam to be his companion, worked the ruin of mankind, when they wish to wreak vengeance upon man, the pagan gods invent woman; and it is the first-born of these female creatures, Pandora, who lets loose all the ills of suffering humanity. The Other—she is passivity confronting activity, diversity that destroys unity, matter as opposed to form, disorder against order. Woman is thus dedicated to Evil."[5]

Women as Inferior

Eleanor Commo McLaughlin, a church historian, emphasizes the "evidence is overwhelming that the medieval Christian theological tradition and the symbols that it generated . . . did provide important stimuli and a convenient ideology for the dehumanization of the female sex."[7] Although their work has been buried and silenced until the present women's movement, early feminists were acutely aware of the damaging effects of religious beliefs on the health and welfare of women. In 1857, Sarah M. Grimke declared that "Woman, instead of being elevated by her union with man, which might be expected from an alliance with a superior being, is in reality lowered. She generally loses her individuality, her independent character, her moral being."[7]

Further reacting to the biblical notion that the male was created as a being superior to the female. Grimke expressed her views on the matter. "The idea that man, as man is superior to woman involves an absurdity so gross that I really wonder how any man of reflection can receive it as of divine origin, and I can only account for it by that passion for supremacy which characterizes man as a corrupt and fallen creature."[7]

However absurd the idea, prominent philosophers have wholeheartedly subscribed to the notion of male superiority. Sr. Thomas Aquinas, as a voice of the masculine age, argued that "woman is defective and misbegotten, for the active force in the male seed tends to the production of a perfect . . . masculine sex, while the production of woman comes from a defect in the active force or from some material indisposition . . ."[7]

Woman as Servant

In *The Church and the Second Sex*, Daly has commented that Sr. Thomas shared the commonly held view that women are not quite human. According to Daly, Thomas viewed women as having an intellectual inferiority that necessitated their also having social inferiority. Since women were inferior, their subjection to men was a "natural" state. As Daly explains, Thomas's view was that women should have no autonomy. The most a woman could hope for "even in the best of worlds, would be a kind of eternal childhood, in which she would be subject to man for her own benefit."[8]

Another philosopher, Rousseau, a male supremacist of the worst kind, argued that "since women are made to please men and be useful to them, the entire education of the female should be directed toward that end."[7] Rousseau taught that women "must be subject, all their lives, to the most severe restraint." He believed women should never be permitted, "for a moment to perceive themselves entirely freed from restraint."[7] In elaborating on the need to restrain women, he noted, "There results from this habitual restraint a tractableness which the women have occasion for during their whole lives as they constantly remain either under subjection to the men, or to the opinions of mankind, and are never permitted to set themselves above those opinions."[7]

Rousseau further argued that women should quietly, with a mild disposition, suffer injustice, insults and believe in false religions in order to remain rightfully subjected, pleasing and useful to men. He thought the "criminality" of women's errors would be overlooked by god, since women were too defective to make judgments for themselves.[7]

Aristotle, who argued that man is a political being and that order in a society depended on the determination of what was just, also argued that man alone was fit to command and woman was made to obey. He concluded that women could not be good, in the same sense that man could be good.[7]

There is no end to the misogynous beliefs expressed in religious and philosophical writings. Historical writings of males repeatedly set forth arguments that women are defective, inferior and have no sense of justice. One final example from a philosopher provides reason enough for women to examine the nature of the politics of care to determine why patriarchal dominance has depleted the human capacity to care. In declaring that the "fundamental fault of the female character is that it has no sense of justice." Schopenhauer noted that "The weakness of their reasoning faculty also explains why it is that women show more sympathy for the unfortunate than men do, and so treat them with more kindness and interest; and what it is that . . . they are inferior to men in point of justice, and less honorable and conscientious."[7]

Here, Schopenhauer is really finding fault with women's capacity to care and is attributing this capacity to their ineffective reasoning ability or their intellectual inferiority. Religious teachers and philosophers have overwhelmingly argued that it was woman's nature to be kind, gentle, loving, and nurturing, but many at the same time argued that this behavior was an outgrowth of their defective nature.

The early feminist philosopher, Mary Wollstonecraft, expressed an acute sense of injustice when she proclaimed in reaction to misogynous views about women: "How grossly do then insult us who thus advise us only to render ourselves gentle, domestic brutes!"[9] In acknowledging that women had been socially and politically conditioned into a state of inferiority, she identified the influence of men as the major cause of women's inability to grow beyond this state. In her words, "I shall only insist that men have increased that inferiority till women are almost stuck below the standard of rational creatures."[9] Wollstonecraft was indignant about the fallacious and hate-filled ideas that enslaved the minds and bodies of the female sex.

Power of Structured Misogyny

Misogynous beliefs did not originate with women. They originated with men and have served the purpose of causing both women and men to hold deep-seated misogynous notions about women.[2,3,6] The power in these structured beliefs has led to longstanding hatred and denigration of women and to the societal worship of the male phallus. Just as patriarchal religions center around the worship of a male god, our societal institutions exist to honor and worship male performance. Male dominance and the worship of males go hand in hand.[2,3,4] Daly has accurately labeled our society phallocratic, noting that "patriarchy is itself the prevailing religion of the entire planet."[3]

STRUCTURED MISOGYNY IN THEORY

In analyzing existing psychological theory, there is clear evidence that patriarchal systems of belief measure all human existence from the standpoint of the existence or lack of existence of male genitals. Within these systems of belief, women are, of course, found lacking and appear as mutilated defectives horrifying to the human mind and eye.[2,3,8] This picture of woman stands out blatantly in psychological theories in common use by nurses.

Reuther gives Freud the distinction of being "the founder of the sexist perversion of psychoanalytic interpretation."[2] Although in my opinion this is quite true where psychoanalytic interpretation is concerned, in his theory Freud was merely repeating the basic misogynous beliefs espoused by male religious leaders and philosophers. His limited vision, influenced solely by a society that embraced only misogynous beliefs, could not conceive of woman as being anything other than what men had always thought her to be.

Freud accepted without questioning the ancient and philosophic view that women are biologically defective. For Freud, this limits and conditions the entire course of women's psychological development, and keeps women from reaching higher realms of intelligence and moral discipline. Freud's theory explicitly states that male genital characteristics are the normative foundation for full humanity against which norm women are found to be defined as deprived or "castrated." Freud even goes to what I consider the ridiculous length, seldom questioned by nurses, to state that very young girls realize their "castrated" state and feel inferior because of it.[2,4]

Freud's misogynistic beliefs entirely pervade his theory, presenting a view of women's lifelong development as a no-win, completely inferior prospect. According to Freud, once the young girl realizes her "castrated" condition, she turns away from the mother to the more powerful father in hopes of receiving a penis, which the father has and the mother lacks. The young girl's psychic development thereafter is a frustrated quest to receive from males, most often the father, husband, or a son, the potency that she has been deprived of by nature.[2,4]

Freud's "Normal" Woman

According to Freud, the lifelong quest to make up for their inherent deficiency leads women to three possible types of development. The first two types Freud views as pathological. The third, which is pathological, Freud views as "normal." First, women can withdraw into neurosis or resentment, burying feelings of depravation as a refusal to relate to others to any great extent.

Second, women can refuse to accept the fact of their "castrated" nature and organize their personality around their clitoris, or rudimentary penis, which gave them pleasure and was the basis of their oedipal desires as an infant. The second option Freud called the masculinity complex, which gives rise to a woman's attempt to emulate men and to pretend that they have exactly the same nature as men. Freud viewed the aggressive, professional or intellectual woman as this type of infantile, clitoral woman, her behavior arising from her refusal to accept her "castrated" nature. Freud viewed women who entered psychoanalysis as doing so because of their penis envy, seeking to obtain from the psychoanalyst-father what their own fathers had failed to give them.

The third option Freud sees as possible for women's lifelong development reflects the most subtle/blatant and damaging form of misogyny. The woman accepts the fact of her "castrated" inferior and defective nature, and essentially worships her father, husband, son and other men because they have male genitals. For Freud, this type of personality development is "normal," and follows a course of gradual acceptance by the woman of her biological fate. The woman then resigns herself to her secondary and dependent destiny, wasting her personal life in pursuit of having a man of one sort or another. Freud's description of this course of development, while ridiculous in the extreme and, indeed perverse as Reuther calls it, reflects ancient patriarchal myths about feminine sexuality.

According to Freud, the "normal" woman must shift the source of her desires from the active libido in the clitoris to the vagina, where she awaits penetration by the male as the source of her feminine fulfillment. This shift requires giving up her drive to grow and develop her potential and demands her acceptance that her true biological destiny requires that she remain a passive, dependent orifice that waits for masculine activity and penetration. It is in making this regressive, growth-denying shift that the woman finally achieves compensation for her deprivation—a baby.[2] As Ruether points out in analyzing Freud's position, of course, not just any baby will do. What women desire primarily is a boy baby—the penis-baby through which they possess, vicariously in their son, what they have been deprived of in themselves. To produce a girl-baby is to create just another mutilation.[2]

Freud's views about penis-babies are similar to those of Sr. Thomas Aquinas, who believed that the male seed tended to reproduce itself only, that is, only male children were normal reproductive products. If a child was born female, it was because something drastic had gone wrong.[2] When analyzed, Freud's theory is a form of structured misogyny having tremendous power over the shaping of modern social thought and action. Such theories should be viewed as having raped the minds and spirits of nurses and of women, generally serving no good purpose for women, only the purpose of forcing women to worship males and their phallocentric ideations, institutions and practices, however demeaning these are to women.

Perpetuating Misogynous Beliefs in Nursing

Curricula in schools of nursing all over this country perpetuate misogynous views of women by teaching the theories similar to those analyzed in this article and then expect nurses to consider themselves educated, self-confident and qualified enough to help women achieve healthy minds and bodies. As I have observed, most nurses who have master's or doctoral degrees in the field of mental health and psychiatric nursing were taught to accept, absorb and believe that Freudian and neo-Freudian theories made sense. To illustrate the damage to nurses, most undergraduate programs in nursing encourage students to read the works of Maslow because he has written a good deal about so-called "health" and self-actualization. Following is a quote that speaks volumes about Maslow's real beliefs on the health of women. In writing about healthy individuals, Maslow says it is essential for a woman:

> to be able to adore a man, to look up to him as once she looked up
> to her father, to be able to lean on him, to be able to trust him, to feel

him to be reliable, to feel him to be strong enough so that she can feel precious, delicate, dainty, and so that she can trustfully struggle down on his lap and let him take care of her and the babies, and the world, and everything else outside the home. This is especially so when she's pregnant, or when she's raising small infants and children. Then she most needs a man around to take care of her, to protect her, and to mediate between her and the world. . . . If she cannot perceive in him the ultimate, eternal, B-masculine qualities, she must be profoundly and deeply unhappy as any woman without a man must be.[10]

Maslow's indirectly expressed hatred and ambivalence toward women is more clearly evident when he writes about the nature of man's "love" for woman:

Now the truth is that any woman, especially to the perceptive eye, to the sensitive man, to the more aesthetic man, to the more intelligent man, to the more healthy man, can be seen as a B-way, with B-cognition, however much a prostitute or a psychopath or a gold digger or a hateful murderess or a witch she may be. The truth is that at some moments she will suddenly flip into her goddess-like aspect, most especially when she's fulfilling those biological functions that men see as basically female, nursing, feeding, giving birth, taking care of children, cleaning the baby, being beautiful, sexually exciting, etc.[10]

As the reader should note, Maslow says nothing derogatory about men. He uses no words that might cause the imagination to conceive of a man as ever having a fault. According to Maslow's view, men are obviously nearly perfect all the time. He strongly emphasizes that men must overlook the basic nature of evil in women in order to "love" them. This comes from a theorist who argues that human nature is basically and intrinsically good. Maslow's belief about women as being all evil (or good and saintlike in rare moments) aptly describes the contradictory images of the nurse. Nurses are commonly portrayed as witches, bitches and whores or saintly angels of mercy. (See "The Public Image of the Nurse" in this issue.)

Without careful efforts to point out the misogynous content inherent in their words, I believe educators in nursing must refuse to each ideas, such as Maslow's and Freud's, that are grossly denigrating to women. If nurses are to effectively analyze the politics of care, if they are to change education and practice in a favorable direction, all practitioners in nursing must become increasingly aware of the subtle ways hatred of women is communicated in patriarchal institutions and settings. Certainly, huge amounts of nurses' time and energy need to be devoted to research designed to analyze and correct misogynous ideas inherent in theories and bodies of knowledge widely used by professionals and consumers of health care. Until nurses have begun this research task, we will not have taken the first step toward an adequate resolution of the problems surrounding the politics of care in this country.

LIVING POWER OF WORDS: IDEAS AND MYTHS

Religion, philosophy and theory create myths and ideas that shape human experience. The political and social roles of language and ideas have not received much attention in nursing literature. However, language and ideas are alive, having constant effects and shaping the lives of individuals, nations and the human race. Lewis Thomas reminds us that "the gift of language is the single human trait that marks us all genetically, setting us apart from all the rest of life." He further notes: "Language, once it comes alive, behaves like an active, mobile organism." Like life itself, "parts of it are always being changed, by a ceaseless activity."[11]

The energy to maintain psychological and social life comes from words and ideas that give meaning and nourishment to life. To understand the politics of any society, the living words and the language of the people are of primary importance. Without language the words that renew the energies of life, we literally die spiritually with much disease caused by the blockage of free-flowing psychic and physical energy necessary for maintaining a healthy organism.[11,12]

The myth of male superiority, of phallic superiority, is alive and survives in religion and in major theories or systems of belief purporting to be scientific in origin.[2,3] Religion is, of course, supposed to be based on meaningful myths, but the substance of scientific theory is assumed to go beyond mythical supposition and embody truths when possible. Myths often hide truths, and as James Hillman points out, "The myth that is alive is not noticed as mythical and seen through."[12] In a careful analysis of language and ideas, nurses are beginning to see through the myth of phallic superiority, finally beginning to understand most, if not all, of the energy-draining issues sapping the spirits of nurses. Confronting the political nature of the myth of phallic superiority will shed much light on the detrimental ways in which this myth enables men to continue exercising male power over women. Presently, and historically, the psychic and physical health of women has been undermined. The survival of women's psychic and physical health is now at stake more than ever, making it necessary to create new words and ideas that will re-energize women.

We need to know, and to have written in our nursing literature, the effects words and ideas have on our thoughts and behaviors. Then, as women, we can start thinking differently and acting differently. As observed everywhere, in the written word, in films and drama, in verbal conversations, in the real, practical world where nurses live and work, nurses are put down and degraded. The degradation arise from nurses' attachment to and involvement with the cult of true womanhood—defined in our misogynous society as serving, pleasing and seeking approval of males. Nurses are, on the surface, praised, rewarded and given token but subversive gains because of their "womanly" service. Yet that very service and cult works to keep nurses subjugated, powerless and politically impotent. This cult and all the definitions we know of womanhood have grown out of phallic worship.

Men recognize that if they do not use their power (in misogyny) to keep women politically impotent, the balance of power would change and they would lose their privileged position in society. Therefore, men fear change in women, and this fear runs as deep as the misogynous beliefs perpetuated about women in our society.[2,3,4,5,13] Feminist scholars make a good cause supporting the view that men do not want women to become healthy holistically, no longer victims of misogyny, a view having a great deal to do with the politics of care and the issue of whether men have the capacity to care for women. Rich makes it clear that men fear healthy change in women because they think that "in becoming whole human beings, women will cease to mother men, to provide the breast, the lullaby, the continuous attention associated by the infant with the mother. Much male fear . . . is infantilism—the longing to remain the mother's son, to possess a woman who exists purely for him."[6]

Words and ideologies are followed by action, by policy and by the formation of laws and social institutions. The old saying that actions speak louder than words is not really true. Actions are always preceded by words. Actions take shape after words have been through, spoken and written. This is why education is valued. It shapes minds, spirits and actions. Hillman makes the interesting observation that "words, too, burn and become flesh as we speak."[12] If this is true, nurses would do well to spend a good deal of time trying to imagine what the battered, scared and bruised souls and minds of women, our own and that of our neighbor, must look like.

Hillman further elaborates on the power and politics of words:

> We need to recall that we do not just make words up or learn them in school, or ever have them fully under control. Words . . . are powers which have invisible power over us. They are personal presences which have whole mythologies, genders, genealogies . . . histories, and vogues, and their own guarding, blaspheming, creating, and annihilating effects. For words are persons. This aspect of the word transcends their nominalistic definitions and contexts and evokes in our souls a universal resonance. Without the inherence of soul in words, speech would not move us, words would not provide forms of carrying out lives and giving sense to our deaths.[12]

MISOGYNY EXPRESSED IN OPPOSITION TO WOMEN'S EDUCATION AND DEVELOPMENT

The power and political use of words cannot be overemphasized. Men have always been aware of this power. It is a power they have never wanted women to gain.[13] Thus their strong historical opposition to women obtaining an education that would enlighten their minds and enable them to create their own thoughts and words, thoughts and words not originating with men.

Virginia Woolf tells of a woman who applied for admission to the Royal College of Surgeons in Edinburgh in 1869. At the time, medical students gathered in a group, howling with laughter, singing merry songs of ridicule. Of course, the male authorities did not permit women to enter their college.[13]

Where attitudes toward women are concerned, the times have not changed much since 1869. In today's society, women who choose to enter male-dominated sciences are cruelly insulted, and males overtly attempt to destroy their psychological health. Evelyn Fox Keller reports on her experiences while trying to obtain a degree in physics at Harvard. She was in essence told that she was not "good enough" to be in the field. She was watched constantly, psychologically and socially isolated, subjected to rude male laughter, to "unmitigated provocation, insult and denial."[14]

In my analysis, Keller remained sane only because she was a strong woman. Both the educated and uneducated men at Harvard displayed their incapacity to care for this woman and her potential. Instead they did all they could possibly do to drive her insane. The men overtly denied her perceptions, her values and her ambitions, forcing her into a state of complete demoralization. From her experiences with male hatred and hostility, Keller concluded that if she had been more politically and socially astute she would not have persisted in searching for affirmation from males who had no capacity to give her any.[14]

Documentation of Misogyny

As women in the male sciences begin to relate and document their experience, the horrors women confront in the male sciences reveal themselves to have no end. One such experience is related by Naomi Weisstein, in telling of her experiences in experimental psychology. She reports that this male-dominated profession considered her research activity an "outrageous violation of the social order" and "against all the laws of nature" only because she was a woman. On the day of her arrival at graduate school, one of the "star" male professors, while puffing on his pipe, told her that women do not belong in graduate school.[14] Following the role model of the professor, the male graduate students "as if by prearranged signal, then leaned back in their chairs, puffed on their newly bought pipes, nodded, and assented. "Yeah," "Yeah," said the male graduate students. "No man is going to want you. No man wants a woman who is more intelligent than he is . . . You're out of your *natural* role. You are no longer feminine."[14]

Weisstein concluded that "the most painful of the appalling working conditions for women in science is the peculiar kind of social-sexual assault women sustain . . . When feminists say that women are treated as sex objects, we are compressing into a single, perhaps rhetorical phrase, an enormous area of discomfort, pain, harassment, and humiliation."[14]

As Weisstein's experience illustrates, the misogyny of the language in psychological theories does not remain in theoretical form, it is alive and overtly manifested in the behavior of male psychologists.[2,3,4] As Weisstein further relates:

I have been in too many professional meetings where the "joke" slide was a woman's body, dressed or undressed. A woman in a bikini is a favorite with past . . . presents of psychological associations. Hake showed such a slide in his presidential address to the Midwestern Psychological Association, and Harlow, past president of the American Psychological Association, has a whole set of such slides, which he shows at the various colloquia to which he is invited. This business of making jokes at women's bodies constitutes a primary social-sexual assault. The ensuing raucous laughter expresses the shared understanding of what is assumed to be women's primary function—to which we can always be reduced. Showing pictures of nude and sexy women insults us: it puts us in our place. You may think you are a scientist, but what you are is an object for our pleasure and amusement. Don't forget it.[14]

THE POLITICS OF CARE AND FEMINIST CONSCIOUSNESS

Coming to intellectual and emotional grips with the politics of care means coming to grips with the damage done to women by the political use of misogynous ideas commonly expressed in male myths, scientific theories and male behavior. In a book entitled *For Her Own Good: 150 Years of the Experts' Advice to Women*, Barbara Ehrenreich and Deirdre English carefully examine the nature of advice given to women by professional experts. These authors document their conclusions that the advice of professional experts has been most damaging to women. They provide clear evidence that "the male professional hoarded up his knowledge as a kind of property, to be dispensed to wealthy patrons or sold on the market as a commodity. His goal was not to spread the skills of healing, but to concentrate them within the elite interest group he represented."[15]

Ehrenreich and English place special emphasis on the fact that medicine defined women as "sick" because they had a uterus and ovaries and then set out to reinforce that "sickness" by exploiting women with the medical treatments they dispensed that actually induced illness and kept them physically and psychologically less powerful.[3,15] At the present time, this making of sick women is a social problem of massive proportions.[3,15] With feminists questioning the saneness and rationality of this approach of women's health, members of the traditional health professions are losing their credibility as health professionals and as a result will ultimately lose all of their power over the minds and bodies of women as they lose the power granted by their profession.

Men Caring for Women

In analyzing the historical evidence, it is clear that the traditional "health" professions have not demonstrated that they are interested in health.[3,15] Since these professions have been dominated by males, we must raise the serious question of whether men have the capacity to care for women at all. There is an abundant amount of evidence indicating that this capacity is limited, if it does exist. We must therefore question man's ability to change the position of women in this system.

In maintaining a close and longstanding relationship to medicine, psychiatry, gynecology, psychology and many other male-dominated groups in the health field, which are based on the noncapacity to care for women, nursing has done great damage to itself, destroying its potential for power, prostituting the practice of nursing and killing the moral consciousness of nurses. In clinging these male-dominated groups in various interdisciplinary relationships, nurses have swallowed whole and live out the mythical beliefs and realities inherent in the cult of true womanhood as defined by men. Women in the nursing profession have not begun to examine the destructive nature of these relationships.

Rich clearly explains why women can no longer ignore the power in and the detrimental effects of patriarchal thinking:

> patriarchal man is in dangerous confusion about his "private" interest. For centuries, patriarchy has maintained itself by asking what was good for males, has assumed male norms and values as universal ones, has allowed the differences of "otherness," the division of male and female consciousness, to become a terrifying dissociation of sensibility. The idea of woman exists at a strangely primitive level in the male psyche. She remains, for all his psychological self-consciousness, the object-figure on which can be projected all that man does not understand, all that he needs, all that he dreads, in his own experience. (Erich Neumann. . . . went so far as to say that man's consequent fear and hatred of woman has been so deep that were it not for his sexual need for women they could have been extirpated as a group.) Denying his own feminine aspects, always associating his manhood with his ability to possess and dominate women, man the patriarch has slowly, imperceptibly, over time, achieved a degree of self-estrangement, self-hatred, and self-mutilation which is coming to have almost irreversible effects on human relationships and on the natural world.[6]

Man's projection of self-hatred and self-mutilation onto woman actually results in the real mutilation and destruction of women. Indeed, power structures and relationships built on male misogyny are highly destructive for both women and men. Identification with these structures and relationships has resulted in the fragmentation of women's power, interests, work, health, and capacity to care for self and for other women. Despite fragmentation, women (especially those who identify with the cult of "true womanhood" as defined by men) still strive for the graspable illusion of power, rather than the difficult to obtain "real thing" by attaching to men as the sustainers, supporters or assistants of men in accomplishing men's work.

Nurses as "Token Torturer"

In such a role in the male-dominated "health" professions, nurses have a very serious problem of being publicly identified as the "token torturers" of other women. Daly elaborates on this problem:

> The medical employment of women as token torturers as evident in the use of nurses, physiotherapists, and token women doctors. In the field of body-gynecology, the nurse, trained to be totally obedient to the Olympian Doctor, functions as the proximate and visible agent of painful and destructive treatment. Nurses shave women about to give birth and give enemas to women in labor. It is they who give injections and it is they who withhold pain medication begged for by the patient. Programmed not to answer women's questions, they sometimes magnify suffering by unreasonable silence and degrading non-answers . . . most unpleasant procedures which nurses perform . . . are done while the woman is awake and aware of being hurt, whereas the deepest wounding—cutting in surgery—which is performed by doctors is done under anesthesia. This . . . within the hospital situation most procedures experienced as painful by women, whereas the doctors' actions—prescribing drugs which often have harmful effects, issuing orders from on high—are often not directly perceived. The nurse, then, functions as token torturer in the primary sense of the term token that is, an outward indication or expression. She is both weapon and shield for the divine doctor.[3]

184

Thoughtful, insightful and perceptive feminists are finally seeing through the myths that surround abusive medical practices directed toward women patients. As Daly notes, the rituals of medicine are more often than not sadistic and "the processions of necrophilic medicine are endless."[3]

Fragmentation and the illusion of power on the part of many nurses who have accepted the patriarchal structure of their profession have created a wide gulf that generally separates them from the experiences of women. In other words, nurses who have struggled to become "professionals" have by that patriarchal definition of "professional" been forced to leave behind their true identity as women. Many nurses are deaf, dumb and blind to the needs of women; nurses are often cruel and abusive to women and to other nurses. In pursuit of male approval, this group of nurses will lie to, cheat, steal from and kill the spirits of women in order to support and serve the purposes of male professionals. The fact that many nurses do this out of ignorance does not excuse the guilt of participating in destructive behavior originating with males.

THE PERSONAL IS POLITICAL

The liberation and freeing of women from the grip of structured misogyny is an idea whose time has come. The liberation and freeing has psychological and physical dimensions. The psychological includes personal and spiritual components of being; the physical encompasses political and social factors forming limiting boundaries around the public and private activities of women. All of these problematic facets serve to restrict and inhibit the being of women.[3]

Since the destruction of the mental and physical health of women is constant in our society, it is time all nurses, from licensed, practical nurses to nurses with doctorates, to seize the opportunity for beginning their journey into an exploration of the politics of care. Where nurses are concerned, issues surrounding nursing and health care generally cannot be separated from feminist issues. For the individual, the need for health and nursing care and efforts to obtain these boil down to a personal concern. Women have coined the phrase that the personal is political.[16–18] This phrase and its meaning have tremendous implication for the social stance most likely to be successful in analyzing the politics of care.

Identifying the personal as political is a means of providing women with an avenue for examining the personal aspects of women's lives in political terms. The necessity of taking this approach seems obvious, since women's experience has been centrally concerned with the personal, private dimensions of human life. Within patriarchal society, women have been largely excluded from public life, left primarily to care for the personal concerns of men and children within the context of the family. As illustrated in this article, when women have engaged in the activities of public life, they have been grossly ignored, negated and devalued. Operating within the realm of the personal, it is only logical that women's devalued personal world be subjected to political analysis, opening a door to an extensive examination of how that which is personal provides the foundations of political and social superstructures controlling the lives of women, a control that remains mostly uninfluenced by women.

The Myth of Professionalization

In a mad rush of confusion, confronting contradictions and illusions, we nurses have mistakenly pursued the myth of professionalism, hoping that the public achievement of this state would provide us with the prestige, recognition and acceptance traditionally accorded male professionals. In our haste to imitate male professionals, we have overlooked the political implications of our personal pursuits. Writing some time ago, Woolf raised the question of why women would want to enter male professions or become like male professionals. She noted that the professions made the men who practiced them "possessive, jealous of any infringement of their rights, and highly combative if anyone dares dispute them."[13] Moreover, Woolf was not unaware of the egotism and greed that characterize educated men who spend their time in "committee rooms, soliciting favours, assuming a mask of reverence to cloak ridicule."[16]

Nurses would do well to follow Woolf's example of seriously considering the effect the professions have on those who practice them. Women are just now beginning to look at the effects the professions have had on society, and the conclusions are not very praiseworthy. Certainly from a political standpoint, we nurses, in our efforts to model our profession after male-defined concepts have overlooked the extent to which this model has repeatedly negated the value of nursing and its scientific/artistic development. As nurses we have grossly overlooked the fact that in a patriarchal society the means of nurturing the personal development of women's potential is not a priority. Patriarchal religion, philosophy and theory have created the reality of women's personal world and personal views of themselves, yielding women almost totally powerless in both personal and political experience.

For the care and development of women's potential to become a reality, all women must learn to care first for women. In doing this we will not model ourselves or our profession after male ideations or standards. I have illustrated the fact that males and male professionals have only a limited capacity to care for women, if they have this capacity at all. This male limitation must be understood before we can begin to get a clear picture of the meaning of the politics of care.

NURSING—THE TURNING POINT

For many years we have heard that nursing is at the crossroads. Nursing never seems to get over being at a crossroads. Indeed, nursing has been at a crossroads many times, but instead of taking a new road, leaders in the profession always choose to continue bearing the burden of continuing to live out the subservient role under the patriarchal system, rather than taking a new road that can lead beyond patriarchy. Nursing is no longer at a crossroads. It is at a turning point. It needs to turn away from being the "token torturer" of itself and other women. It needs to turn toward the health awaiting women in a woman-defined, woman-created world that lies beyond patriarchal ideas and institutions.[2,6]

Finally, after more than a century of existence, the nursing profession needs to become a self-directing, honorable profession, unashamed of its efforts and its aims, rightly divining the word of truth where it can be found. In order to become self-directing, honorable and unashamed of searching for its own truth, nursing must shed its petty and childish fears of feminism and begin to embrace the powerful knowledge and insights to be gained from feminist literature. I believe nursing cannot become self-directing or effective in the politics of care without embracing feminism and all it stands for.

Validating Nursing Experience

If nursing is to become self-directing and effective in the politics of care, nurses cannot continue to identify with male-dominated professions for the reasons I have already outlined, ignoring the problems of real, live nurses and the problems of women in general. Rich speaks of this issue:

> For if, in trying to join the common world of men, the professions molded by a primarily masculine consciousness, we split ourselves off from the common life of women and deny our female heritage and identify in our work, we lose touch with our real powers and with the essential condition for all fully realized work: community.
>
> Feminism begins but cannot end with the discovery by its individual of self-consciousness as a woman. It is not, finally, even the recognition of her reasons for anger, or the decision to change her life, go back to school, leave a marriage . . . Feminism means finally that we renounce our obedience to the fathers and recognize that the world they have described is not the whole world. Masculine ideologies are the creation of masculine subjectivity; they are neither objective, nor value-free, nor inclusively "human." Feminism implies that we recognize fully the inadequacy for us, the distortion, of male-created ideologies, and that we proceed to think, and act, out of that recognition.[6]

When analyzed, medical ideology and all the ideologies of the traditional health professions are masculine ideologies. As such, they negate the very existence of nursing as a separate and valid profession with much of value to offer society, a service that goes beyond mere treatment of disease to the provision of needed care for the health of people.

In accepting the token generosity of fatherly figures in the medical profession and in other fields of male scholarship, nurses negate the validity of their own experiences, thereby losing the power they might have by identifying with the needs and concerns of all women. In the future, nursing practice should focus all of its attention on validating the experiences of women. Women comprise 70 percent of the work force in all health care settings.[19] Since women risk their health by going to male professionals, nurses have the large task of warning women that this risk is real and dangerous. The professional obligation of the nurse as an advocate of the woman client is that of explaining the risks involved, and helping her to safeguard her health by finding competent and reliable practitioners who will meet her needs for humane care. From a sound political and ethical standpoint, nurses cannot avoid undermining the unwarranted confidence that women tend to place in unscrupulous professionals.

Nurses Caring for Nurses

In examining the politics of care, nurses should also examine their own profession. The nursing profession is divided into various levels of women workers. To date, organized nursing has done little toward studying the specific problems of these various groups of women workers. Instead, nurses support the patriarchal phenomena of divide and conquer, which continues to succeed in splitting and fragmenting the efforts of all nurses. Nurses remain psychologically and socially isolated from one another. Their loyalties remain false and misplaced.

The hostility nurses feel toward other nurses is overtly expressed. Nurses have never examined the male origins of this hostility, which arises from all the misogynous beliefs held about women. Men have despised the work of women, devaluing it and giving it no real place in history. Taking place largely as a form of servitude, women's work and its value have gone unnoticed. Modeling themselves after males, women also devalue the work of other women, particularly women who are viewed as "the other" because of different levels of educational preparation.

It is truly a shameful thing that professionally prepared nurses cannot care for and value the lives and experiences of nurses' aides, practical nurses, associate degree and diploma graduates. It is shameful that no connection or sense of community exists between these groups of women. If nurses would begin to care for other nurses, the profession would have more than enough power necessary for controlling its practice and its destiny. The effective use of a caring kind of politics will not become a reality until nurses begin to make meaningful connections with the lives of other nurses and women, establishing community of sharing, caring. This is the type of politics that is feared by the patriarchy and that can be personally and publicly effective in overcoming the damages wrought by the same patriarchy.

The power, the politics, and the practice of feminism are devoted to the preservation of human life and to its nourishment. Feminism is devoted to the preservation of the earth's resources as a necessity for the preservation of human life and health. These goals should be the goals of my politics of care. And these should be the goals of nursing practice born now and in the future. Exploring, examining, embracing and employing the ideas, beliefs, values and actions of feminism can provide nurses with a new and vital source of energy—energy that is absolutely necessary for healthy performance in women's lives. Women nurses are women first. If we consistently remember this, accepting our heritage and strengths as women, our politics of care can begin.

REFERENCES

1. Thompson, W. I. (1978). *Darkness and scattered light* (p. 44). Garden City, NY: Anchor Press.
2. Ruether, R. R. (1975). *New woman new earth: Sexist ideologies and human liberation* (pp. xi, 138, 140). New York: The Seabury Press.
3. Daly, M. Gyn/Ecology: (1978). *The metaethics of radical feminism* (pp. 39, 103–106, 274, 276–277). Boston: Beacon Press.

4. Bianchi, E. C., & Ruether, R. R. (1976). *From machismo to mutuality: Woman-Man liberation* (pp. 12–13). New York: Paulist Press.

5. de Beauvoir, S. (1976). *The second sex*, trans. and ed. H. M. Parshley. New York: Alfred A. Knopf.

6. Rich, A. (1979). *On lies, secrets, and silence* (pp. 110–111, 207, 221). New York: W. W. Norton & Co.

7. Osborne, M. L. et al. (1979). *Woman in western thought* (pp. 41–45, 69, 99, 106, 107, 113, 114, 214). New York: Random House.

8. Daly, M. (1968). *The church and the second sex* (p. 93). New York: Harper & Row, Publishers.

9. Wollstonecraft, M. (1971). *A vindication of the rights of woman* (pp. 55, 70). New York: W. W. Norton & Co.

10. Maslow, A. H. (1964). *Religion, values and peak experiences* (pp. 107–108, 110). New York: Penguin Books.

11. Lewis, T. (1975). *The lives of a cell* (pp. 105–106). New York: Bantam Books.

12. Hillman, J. (1975). *Re-Visioning psychology* (pp. 9, 155). New York: Harper & Row, Publishers.

13. Woolf, V. (1938). *Three guineas* (p. 66). New York: Harcourt, Brace and World.

14. Weisstein, N. Y. (1977). "How Can a Little Girl Like You Teach a Great Big Class of Men? The Chairman said, and Other Adventures of a Woman in Science" in Ruddick, S. and Daniels, P., eds. *Working it out. 23 women writers, artists, scientists, and scholars talk about their lives and work* (pp. 78–91, 242–250). New York: Pantheon Books.

15. Ehrenreich, B., & English, D. (1978). *For her own good: 150 years of experts' advice to women* (p. 30). Garden City, NY: Anchor Press.

16. Koedt, A., Levine, E., & Rapone, A. (Eds.). (1973). *Radical feminism.* New York: Quadrangle.

17. Morgan, R. (1978). *Going too far.* New York: Vintage Books.

18. Firestone, S. (1970). *The dialectic of sex: The case for feminist revolution.* New York: Bantam Books.

19. Hackett, O. P. (1977). "Women and the Health System: A Case Study in Feminist Praxis." *Radical Religion,(3),2* (pp. 36–43).

BIBLIOGRAPHY

Berkin, C. R., & Norton, M. B. (1979). *Women of America: A history.* Boston: Houghton Mifflin Co.

Brownmiller, S. (1975). *Against our will: Men, women and rape.* New York: Simon & Schuster.

Clark, E., & Richardson, H., (Eds.). (1977). *Women and religion.* New York: Harper & Rox, Publishers.

Corea, G. (1977). *The hidden malpractice.* New York: Jove Publications.

Daly, M. (1973). *Beyond God the Father.* Boston: Beacon Press.

David, D. S., & Brannon, R., (Eds.). (1976). *The forty-nine percent majority: The male sex role.* Menlo Park, CA: Addison-Wesley Publishing Co.

DeCrow, K. (1975). *Sexist justice.* New York: Vintage Books.

Dinnerstein, D. (1977). *The mermaid and the minotaur.* New York: Harper & Row, Publishers.

Dworkin, A. (1974). *Woman hating.* New York: E. P. Dutton & Co.

Frankfort, E. (1972). *Vaginal politics.* New York: Bantam Books.

Goldenberg, N. (1979). *Changing of the gods.* Boston: Beacon Press.

Greer, G. (1971). *The female eunuch.* New York: Bantam Books.

Griffin, S. (1979). *Rape: The power of connections.* New York: Harper & Row, Publishers.

Griffin, S. (1978). *Women and nature.* New York: Harper & Row, Publishers.

Lederer, W. (1968). *The fear of women.* New York: Harcourt Brace Jovanovich.

Mackinnon, C. A. (1979). *A sexual harassment of working women.* New Haven, CT: Yale University Press.

Nie, J. (1978). *Seven women: Portraits from the feminist radical tradition.* New York: Penguin Books.

Oakley, M. B. (1972). *Elizabeth Cady Stanton.* New York: The Feminist Press.

Pomeroy, S. B. (1975). *Goddesses, whores, wives and slaves.* New York: Schocken Books.

Ruether, R. (1972). *Literature theology.* New York: Paulist Press.

Sangiuliano, I. (1978). *In her time.* New York: William Morrow & Co.

Sochen, J. (1973). *Movers and shakers: American women thinkers and activists, 1900–1970.* New York: Quadrangle/The New York Times Book Co.

Tolston, A. (1977). *The limits of masculinity.* New York: Harper & Row, Publishers.

PART THREE

HISTORICAL THINKING AND NURSING

*L*iving in a world where rapid change appears to move us ever more rapidly into the future, our perspectives on the past (if we even take time to consider them) are often nostalgic and romanticized. Too often we have been turned off to history by years of childhood spent memorizing dates and events. Dr. Ashley was among a critical mass of nursing scholars who pushed for a renaissance in nursing history in the 1970s. During this period of social change, history, and the recognition of its varying interpretations, became essential to the collective consciousness raising of nursing. As Dr. Ashley advises, "the study of history gives people their identity" (1978, p. 35). Unfortunately her untimely death came a few months before the American Association for Nursing History was created in 1981. After the founding meeting for the association, however, I had the opportunity to speak with the late historian Dr. Teresa Christy. She reflected on the loss of her former student and acknowledged that Jo Ann's work, especially with her critical perspectives on paternalism, had generated debate which had served to renew interest in nursing history across the country. Dr. Christy lamented her death and, like many others in nursing, wondered how different the future might have been had she lived longer than her forty years.

This section contains two papers that reflect on the role of historical thinking. The first paper, "Foundation for Scholarship, Historical Thinking in Nursing," was written for the journal, *Advances in Nursing Science*, and published in 1978. This essay considers the benefits of nurses understanding nursing history and the then current state of historical research and its contribution to theory development. A central theme concerns the need to re-examine nursing history as well as the traditional approaches used in doing research and theory development. Generally remembered as a feminist nursing scholar, this paper reveals Ashley's tendency to take a more eclectic approach in her analysis of nursing history. She cites the contribution of Karl Marx to our understanding of the economic exploitation and class-based struggles in health care. She points out that the disunity within the nursing profession is a result of the ongoing class struggle while referencing the growing stratification in nursing by education and skill level and titles. Citing an increase in professional fragmentation and greater confusion thereby for the public, she cautions that the emergence of new health care workers outside of the field of nursing will intensify the class struggle. While she cites physician assistants and emergency room technicians specifically, in recent years nursing has also felt intense competition with the emergence of institutionally trained workers such as patient care technologists and health care technicians. In addition, nursing has repeatedly struggled with the effects of stratification within nursing, including wage depression. Marked diversity in the gender, racial, and ethnic make-up of the various educational and practice groups also often make attempts to unify and reduce stratification difficult.

Funded by the government as "pressure value" in the face of high unemployment, nursing has often provided multiple access points and opportunities for class mobility, especially from lower to middle class. Encouraged by hospitals and financially supported by federal funds, nursing experienced the rapid growth of the community colleges and associate degree (AD) nursing programs. While AD programs accounted for less than 10 percent of nursing graduates in the mid 1960s, their expansion accounts for the production of over 60 percent of the nursing graduates in the mid 1990s (ANA, 1977; NLN, 1994). This trend epitomizes the growing contradiction between desire for exclusive control of educational access by nursing and inclusive unity of a highly stratified labor force. Long viewed as a hallmark of professionalism, control over entry into the labor force has yet remained a conundrum for nursing.

Ashley's consideration of psychological perspectives includes here a less than enthusiastic inclusion of Freud together with an endorsement of psychohistory (Lifton, 1961). Grounded in the clinical practice of psychiatric nursing, Dr. Ashley was drawn to the psychohistorical approach. She endorsed this radical method of historical research as a means to better understand the human experience in periods of great change. She argued that: "(n)urses need to research on the psychohistorical profiles of living nurses; their thoughts and what has served to give meaning to their lives . . . " (Ashley, 1978, p. 35). Through such profiles, Dr. Ashley hoped that young practitioners would be able to make comparisons to their own experience, "a comparison useful in preventing many of the struggles that nurses have lived with in the past" (Ashley, 1978, p.35). As a result, in the late 1970s, Dr. Ashley began an oral history project to study the lives of contemporary nursing. She cites, as the two main purposes of this study, to collect data about the history of nursing as experienced by contemporary nurses and to identify the social, economic, political, and personal factors shaping the lives of those studied. Following the psychohistorical approach proposed by Robert Lifton (1976), but using a feminist framework, from the theories of feminist psychologist Jean Baker Miller (1976) and theorist Rosemary Reuther (1975), Dr. Ashley sought to better understand how nurses dealt with the conflicts arising out of patriarchy and sexism in their personal and professional lives.

The second paper was written a few years earlier as a presentation at the Teachers College, Columbia University Stewart Nursing Research Conference. Entitled, "Myths and Realities of Apprenticeship in Nursing," this paper takes off from her dissertation research to look at the broader context of nursing as women's work, and the role of hospitals in the exploitation of nurses. Similar to her book *Hospitals,*

Paternalism and the Role of the Nurse, this paper introduces the reader to her historical analysis of the rise of the apprenticeship system in nursing.

Dr. Ashley examines several facets of paternalism and nursing: economic, political, legal and social. She cautions that the economic exploitation of nursing students in the apprenticeship system was one means the hospital used to produce cheap labor. Ironically, nursing continues to confront the hospital industry's push for cheaper labor sources. A second facet here concerns the political or legal and legislative efforts to advance and restrain nursing practice. Despite the fact that nursing was one of the three traditional, organized professions in the health field, it received only limited social recognition. Ashley acknowledges that the laws were slow to recognize nurses and more often served to codify their subjugation to medicine. Finally, Ashley turns to the social, including the complexities of ideology and social structures and their effect on gender roles in society.

A central premise of the study is also clear: the general passivity of nursing leadership helped to facilitate the oppression of nurses. Many scholars have taken issue with this perspective, suggesting that it does not allow for consideration of the overall lack of power for women in our society. Ashley is quite harsh on this point, and further suggests that many nursing leaders were blinded as they walked in the shadow of physicians and hospital administrators. Her presentation of nursing history has also been criticized for suggesting that nurses were innocent victims as well as for being perhaps too harsh on nursing leadership generally. Nonetheless, the results of such debate were and are quite beneficial to the profession as a whole: continued discussion on the lessons of history and what nursing could learn as it renewed its struggle to claim professionalism and power.

References

1. ANA. (1977). *Facts about nursing* 76–77. Kansas City: American Nurses Association.

2. Ashley, J. A. (1976). *Hospitals, paternalism and the role of the nurse.* New York: Teachers College Press.

3. Ashley, J. A. (undated) *A Proposal to study the lives of contemporary nurses: An oral history project.*

4. Lifton, R. J. (1976). *The life of the self.* New York: Simon & Schuster.

5. Miller, J. B. (1976). *Toward a new psychology of women.* Boston: Beacon Press.

6. NLN. (1994). *1994 Nursing data Source(Vol 1.): Trends in contemporary nursing education.* New York: NLN Press.

7. Reuther, R. R. (1975). *New women, new earth:Sexist ideologies and human liberation.* New York: The Seabury Press.

Growing into Full Humanness

by Jo Ann Ashley

Growth is change in life.
Life itself is a process of
Deaths and rebirths.
The death of the old must give
Rise to the birth of the new.
In each of us, the force of life
Yearns to bloom and blossom.
Make way for change in your life.
Leave no stone unturned that
Touches the stem of what your life
Can become.

Growing is a process of examining
The past.
It is an effort to know what must
Die
Before conditions for the growth of
The new can be set in us, in our
Society.
The past alone can tell us what not
To do if we are to avoid the stifling
Of new life in us, in our society.

Growth is a sense of openness to what
Is.
It is openness to what will come.
It is openness to what must come if
Realities are to be different for us.
For openness to arise we must know
What we have been,
What we have done.
Our horizons of consciousness must
Expand.
Flexibility is the mark of the open
Woman, the open man.
Openness itself is the mark of the
Fully grown human to full humanness.

Growth is stifled by prejudice, by
Senseless projections.
It is stifled by minds fearful and
Afraid of pure and simple change.
Naked reflection on these things is
The riverbed of truthful, meaningful,
Lifegiving change.

Chapter 11

FOUNDATIONS FOR SCHOLARSHIP

*Historical Research in Nursing**

NEW THEORIES FOR A CHANGING WORLD

Women are beginning to realize that dead and dying theories about the nature of human behavior have failed to say much that is meaningful about the true nature of women. Theories and conceptual frameworks growing out of patriarchal thinking have been damaging to women's health, their self-image and their sense of well-being. But women are finally awakening and beginning to question theories in fields ranging from religion to economics and politics. Although women are not likely to advocate the development of a matriarchal social order, they are no longer willing to go along with the limitations imposed on them by male-dominated traditions. Liberated women want to think freely. They want to develop their own theories to explain the realities of their world and to shape their ideals accordingly.

In *The Modern Researcher*, the authors rightfully point out that facts "are seen through ideas . . . that are not immediately visible and ready to be noted down. They are searched for with a purpose in mind. The facts once ascertained, a mind has to frame a hypothesis to arrive at what is properly called *theory:* a total view of related events."[1]

---

* Reprinted with permission of Aspen Publishers, Inc. © 1980. From *ANS*, (1978), Vol. 1, (no. 1), pp. 25–36.

The mutability of knowledge is well known. Science itself must alter and modify "its interpretations every few years, and on its frontiers hypotheses conflict."[1] The development of women as theorists, scientists and artists will inevitably bring with it vast changes in our thought processes and our perceptions of the world we live in. Already the questions being raised by women have led to the reordering, revision and updating of many ideas and facts.

As an outgrowth of liberating the minds of women and men, future theories will present us with an even more total view of related events than theories of the past have been able to present. In the past, men have been the predominant generators and carriers of ideas, and have been more biased in their development of theories than most of them would care to admit.

Men have not only created ideas, they have used them to give shape and form to our values, beliefs and social organizations. Our legal, economic and political systems with their many constraints on women have also been derived from these biased ideas. The boundaries and limitations placed on women in these systems are the focus of the women's movement and motivate women to seek new knowledge and new interpretations of human behavior and the functioning of society.

In her book *The Human Condition,* Arendt comments on the nature of limitations:

> Limitations and boundaries exist within the realm of human affairs, but they never offer a framework that can reliably withstand the onslaught with which each new generation must insert itself . . . the territorial boundaries which protect and make possible the physical identity of a people, and the laws which protect and make possible its political existence, are of such great importance to the stability of human affairs precisely because no such limiting and protecting principles rise out of the activities going on in the realm of human affairs itself. The limitations of the law are never entirely reliable safeguards against action from without. The boundlessness of action is only the other side of its tremendous capacity for establishing relationships, that is, its specific productivity; this is why the old virtue of moderation, of keeping within bounds, is indeed one of the political virtues par excellence. . . .[2]

Arendt emphasizes that limitations and boundaries are not useful frameworks when social change is in order. This observation is fascinating in relation to women's role in society and especially in relation to the role of the nursing profession. Where nursing is concerned, *the conceptual framework* guiding our development for more than a century has been one of limitations and boundaries. This framework has defined our professional identity, our political existence and relationships in the world of work. The specific productivity of nursing in various economic and social organizations derives from boundaries and limitations which are often not defined by nurses' aspirations, experiences and thinking.

CREATIVITY AS THE FOUNDATION FOR SCHOLARSHIP IN NURSING

It is precisely this framework of boundaries and limitations that the present generation of nursing students and scholars must transcend if we are to develop meaningful theories to guide the expanding horizons of our practice and our persons. Breaking away from old ideas and conceptual frameworks is not an easy task. The leap into what may be new and unfamiliar territory is frightening as well as stimulating. But this leap constitutes the act of creativity required to go forward.

Creativity has not traditionally been the major goal of nursing education, and it has certainly not been a goal in practice settings. It is time, however, for educational programs to make creativity their main objective in teaching, practice and research. The foundations for scholarship in the art and science of nursing must be creativity. Without creativity, we will labor in vain. Without creativity, we will not be fostering scholarship but stagnation, and there will be no new insights to move us forward in thought or in action.

There are several reasons why there has not been more creativity in nursing. First, it is generally recognized that nurses are predominantly women, and women have not been thought capable of really having valuable ideas; society has not expected them to produce ideas and create knowledge. Second, creativity takes time and freedom from excessive pressure and trivial busy work. Many climates in nursing education and practice simply do not provide an atmosphere supportive of creative activity. A jack-of-all trades or a person handy about the house, hospital or clinic does not have the time or energy to concentrate on conceiving new ideas.

Finally, creativity *is not* a totally painless process. Just as bringing a child into the world takes long months of pregnancy and an often painful delivery, the birth of new insights depends on months of pregnant thought followed by disciplined work to give shape and physical form to that thought. In other words, the birth of anything and everything takes time and is accompanied by some pain and some joy. Those people who wish to avoid discomfort are not likely to be found creating anything.

Among works on the process of creativity, May's *The Courage to Create* best describes some of the emotions experienced when a new insight breaks through to consciousness. Here are his own reactions to getting new insights:

> A dynamic struggle goes on within a person between what he or she consciously thinks on the one hand and, on the other, some insight, some perspective that is struggling to be born. The insight is then born with anxiety, guilt, and the joy and gratification that is inseparable from the actualizing of a new idea or vision.
>
> The guilt that is present when this breakthrough occurs has its source in the fact that the insight must destroy something. My [new] insight destroyed . . . [other hypotheses] and . . . destroy [ed] what a number of my professors believed, a fact that caused me some concern. Whenever there is a breakthrough of a significant idea in science or a significant new form in art, the new idea will destroy what a lot of people believe is essential to the survival of their intellectual and spiritual world. This is the source of guilt in genuine creative work. As Picasso remarked, "Every act of creation is first of all an act of destruction."[3]

But May goes on to say, "the main feeling that comes with the breakthrough is one of gratification. We have seen something new. We have the joy of participating in what the physicists and other natural scientists call an experience of 'elegance'."[3] As May so clearly points out in *The Courage to Create*, the essence of creativity is the making of something new. This birth can profoundly disrupt the life of an individual or society. For the advancement of civilization, there are times when it is most appropriate to upset the status quo. Clinging to outdated ideas, values and beliefs is not a constructive use of energy, and it does not provide a sound foundation for scholarship. A creative turning away from what one needs to let go of indicates a healthy responsiveness to the force of life and to changing ideas.

Why should a historian who loves to study and ponder over the past advocate creativity and the avid pursuit of the new as the foundations for scholarship in nursing? History is the study of creative activity in human behavior; studying and understanding the past gives one the courage to create and respond to what is new without fear of losing one's identity with the whole of humanity.

A quote from the historian Williams further explains the purpose and value of historical research in helping people to creatively overcome the binding chains of the past:

> History as a way of learning has one additional value beyond establishing the nature of reality and posing the questions that arise from its complexities and contradictions. It can offer examples of how other . . . [women] faced up to the difficulties and opportunities of their eras. Even if the circumstances are noticeably different, it is illuminating, and productive of humility as well, to watch other . . . [women] make their decisions, and to consider the consequences of their values and methods. If the issues are similar, then the experience is more directly valuable. But in either case the procedure can transform history as a way of learning into a way of breaking the chains of the past.[4]

As another author puts it: "The benefit . . . usually expected of . . . [history] is an enrichment of the imagination that promotes a quick and shrewd understanding of the actions of men in society. Hence the value of historical training to the student of any aspect of man's life and to the worker in any branch of social intelligence."[1] According to this writer, history is the "cornerstone of a liberal education."

CHANGING THE NATURE OF HISTORICAL RESEARCH IN NURSING

Historical research in nursing has, to date, consisted of purely descriptive reporting of data without any conceptual analysis of their meaning for nurses and for society. Creativity in the writing of nursing history has been almost totally lacking. Furthermore, the descriptive reporting of data is all the more meaningless since historical research into nursing has been highly insular with little reference to documents originating outside of our field. Published accounts of the history of nursing cannot be considered history proper. For the most part, they are simple chronological recordings or narratives that do not offer any real explanations or any real understanding of the complexity of our growth and development. Much of the written history of nursing has been used to support illusions that foster false pride. This can be said of the history of medicine as well. There are not, as yet, any accurate histories of the development of the American health care system as a whole.

History is the record of human behaviors, actions, thought and beliefs. These do not occur in a vacuum or in isolation from intellectual ideas shaping a society and its people. History records the struggles of humans to be humans. It tells of wars, prosperity and poverty. History tells of man's inhumanity to man and of woman's inhumanity to woman.

May comments on what he perceives as a prevalent "uninterest in history and the refusal to study it." He associates this lack of interest in history with the need or unconscious wish of Americans to remain innocent. In the words of May:

> To hang on to . . .[a] picture of innocence, you must deny history. For history is the record, among other things, of man's sins and evils, of wars and confrontations of power, and all the other manifestations of man's long struggle toward an enlarged and deepened consciousness.

Hence so many of the new generation turn their backs on history as irrelevant; they do not like it, they are not part of it, they insist we are in a brand-new ball game with new rules. And they are completely unaware that this is the ultimate act of *hubris*.[5]

Within nursing, devaluation of our history is the direct cause of not having any authentic historical studies to give us knowledge to use in deepening the consciousness of our humanity. Our identity has suffered greatly because we have not carefully studied our history and incorporated historical knowledge into theoretical and clinical teachings. Without this knowledge, the foundations of nursing scholarship and practice have indeed been shaky.

Because of the nature of the profession and its holistic approach in dealing with the needs of humanity, nursing has always been and will always be both an art and a science. The devaluation of history has brought shallowness and stagnation to both aspects. Without knowledge of history as a base, the artistic side of any practice field is neglected, ignored and lost sight of almost totally, and the art of nursing is indeed sorely underdeveloped. Without knowing history, one cannot approach knowing truth. Without historical thinking, science can all too easily become a fiction, an illusion, a social lie told with no regard for what is true.

What both nurses and the American public as a whole need are sound, socially enlightening historical studies, studies providing interpretations and analyses of how our health care system developed. Many of today's problems have always existed. The crises we hear so much about in health care are often repeats of history.

To more fully explain such crises and to eliminate their unnecessary recurrence, nursing histories in the future must give us more than isolated facts about nursing and nurses; they must give us meaning and understanding. These histories must explain for the profession and for the public the complex economic and political struggles of nurses and how they relate to other groups, classes and factions within the health care system and within communities and society. Our history in the future must be an intellectual history that examines the ideas and modes of thought shaping the formation of human behaviors and institutions.

THE HISTORIAN AS ARTIST AND SCIENTIST: THINKING HOLISTICALLY

Collecting data and writing intellectual history involve the application of theories and concepts from all fields of knowledge known to humanity. Only with the use of theories and conceptual frameworks can historical data be accurately interpreted; this is the scientific part of the historical researcher's work.

Facts, events, ideas, institutions and societal trends do not speak for themselves, but must be interpreted by a human mind hard at work trying to analyze the continuity, diversity and change involved in the complex interrelationships that characterize human history. In *Historical Thinking*, Tholfsen clearly states the concerns of the historical researcher; these are the dimension of time, the categories of change, continuity and diversity as reflected in human affairs. Within human life the past is connected to the present, and it is the task of the historian to reveal "the nature of man, in his being and becoming in the course of time."[6]

Tholfsen and other male historians tend to see history as the history of man and woman. However, in writing and studying history, it must be kept in mind that the history of man is not the history of woman. Our future histories must distinguish between the two. Much of woman's history is filled with pain and prejudice inflicted upon her by men. The mental reconstruction of this history may well be a somewhat painful task for the female historian who undertakes this reconstruction.

The process will be painful because the historian, through an active use of imagination, actually tries to relive the past. Historians as artists try to feel in body, mind and soul what the people they are studying actually might have felt in their lifetime. A quote from Berlin best describes the artistic side of historical research:

> the historian's activity is an artistic one. Historical explanation is to a large degree arrangement of the discovered facts in patterns which satisfy us because they accord with life—the variety of human experience and activity—as we know it and can imagine it.

. . . This kind of historical explanation is related to moral and aesthetic analysis, in so far as it pre-supposes conceiving of human beings not merely as organisms in space, the regularities of whose behavior can be described and locked in labour saving formulae, but as active, beings pursuing ends, shaping their own and others' lives, feeling, reflecting, imagining, creating, in constant interaction and intercommunication with other human beings; in short, engaged in all the forms of experience that we understand because we share in them, and do not view them purely as external observers.[7]

The historian cannot be narrowly scientific because the recreating, reliving and writing about the past constitute nothing less than a work of art. Another reference to Berlin provides a beautiful explanation of this process:

Capacity for understanding people's characters, knowledge of ways in which they are likely to react to one another, ability to "enter into" their motives, their principles, the movement of thoughts and feelings (and this applies no less to the behavior of masses or to the growth of cultures)—these are the talents that are indispensable to historians, but not . . . to natural scientists.[7]

Nurses should make excellent historians since many of the artistic talents necessary for the making of great historians are also required to make a great nurse. The heart and core of nursing is understanding and feeling for others; these are the essence of the historian's work as well. In an integrated, holistic fashion, both nurse and historian must be skillful in the creative use of intellect and feeling, and both must be artists.

THE USE OF THEORY IN HISTORICAL RESEARCH: SUGGESTED STUDIES

Among other things, history deals with the social, the political and the economic. The use of theories in each of these fields is, therefore, essential in the analysis of historical data. The historian must use old, new and emerging theories and concepts to explain human behavior and to explain the functioning or nonfunctioning of institutions.

It is common knowledge that our health care system is and has been an industry since the turn of the century. It is an economic enterprise, and a lot of money is exchanged in the marketplace of medical care delivery. In this system of capitalistic enterprise, profits are made from the continuing existence of much sickness and disease. People are literally being made mentally and physically sick by this system. This inhumane development is directly related to economic profit. If people in our society were well, happy and relatively healthy, our present health care system would collapse because no one would be making any profits from diseased humanity. Many, if not most, of our past and present problems are purely economic. To understand them fully, we must utilize economic theories.

The theories of Marx are particularly relevant to the history of nursing. It was Marx who came up with the insight that all of history is a history of class struggles. It was Marx who devoted his research and his life to efforts to free oppressed working classes from the miseries of capitalist domination. Since nurses have historically been cast into the role of the subordinate working class or productive force within health care settings, a Marxist interpretation of our struggles and difficulties is imperative for providing new understanding of our plight in the world of work.

A Marxist interpretation of nursing history and the history of the American health care system would also shed light on the dehumanization and disintegration observable within this system. Williams comments interestingly on the appropriate use of Marx's theories in explaining developments in our society:

Americans have never confronted Karl Marx himself. We have never confronted his central theses about the assumptions, the costs, and the nature of capitalist society. We have never confronted his central insight that capitalism is predicated upon an overemphasis and exaltation of the individualistic, egoistic half of man functioning in a marketplace system that overrides and crushes the social, humanitarian half of man. We have never confronted his perception that capitalism is based upon a definition of man in the marketplace that defines the dialogue between men as a competitive struggle for riches and power. And we have never confronted his argument that capitalism cannot create a community in which how much men produce and own is less important than what they make, less important than their relationships as they produce and distribute those products, less important than what they are as men, and less important than how they treat each other.[8]

With our present health care system causing almost more problems than it cures, we must take Marx seriously and carry out historical studies that will explain more fully the damage done to humanity by this capitalistic system. Some of Marx's own thoughts help explain the historical development of class struggles within the nursing profession and medical hierarchy. He wrote:

The history of all hitherto existing society is the history of class struggles.

Freeman and slave, patrician and plebeian, lord and serf, guildmaster and journeyman, in a word, oppressor and oppressed, stood in constant opposition to one another, carried on an uninterrupted, now hidden, now open fight, a fight that each time ended, either in a revolutionary reconstitution of society at large, or in the common ruin of the struggling classes.

In the earlier epochs of history, we find almost everywhere a complicated arrangement of society into various orders, a manifold gradation of social rank. In ancient Rome we have patricians, knights, plebeians, slaves; in the Middle Ages, feudal lords, vassals, guildmasters, journeymen, apprentices, serfs; and in almost all of these particular classes, again, other subordinate gradations.

The modern bourgeois society that has sprouted from the ruins of feudal society has not done away with class antagonisms. It has only established new classes, new conditions of oppression, new forms of struggle in place of the old ones.[9]

This analysis of class struggle describes the American health care system almost perfectly. The elaborate social rankings within medicine, nursing and the emerging paramedical profession can scarcely be comprehended by the public. Consumers and workers alike seldom question the hierarchy and the confusion and competition associated with it. Utilizing economic theories in historical research can lead to an understanding of the damaging effects of this hierarchical health care system.

Within the nursing profession, the various groups or levels of practitioners behave as if they were separate classes, classes constantly struggling and competing for a recognized place in society or the marketplace. The development of physician assistants, emergency technicians and other groups will only intensify these struggles, making the health field even more complex, costly and confusing than it already is to the public.

The lack of unity we hear so much about within nursing is really an outgrowth of class struggle. A historical understanding of these struggles and the political and economic purpose they serve can help us overcome the conflicts we have about them. In addition, utilizing economic theories can help nurses overcome the brainwashing they have been subjected to by economic and social systems that pay them poorly and treat them badly.

From a psychological standpoint, oppression and the brainwashing that accompanies it cause great harm to humans. Nurses have not escaped this kind of damage. There is a need for historical studies that will help nurses analyze and better understand just what has been done to their concept of themselves as persons and as productive humans.

Brown discusses the "disease called man" in his book on psychoanalytic interpretations of history:

The doctrine that all men are mad appears to conflict with a historical perspective on the nature and destiny of man: it appears to swallow all cultural variety, all historical change, into a darkness in which all cats are gray. But this objection neglects the richness and complexity of the Freudian theory of neurosis.

... it is a Freudian theorem that each individual neurosis is not static but dynamic. It is a historical process with its own internal logic. Because of the basically unsatisfactory nature of the neurotic compromise, tension between the repressed and repressing factors persists and produces a constant series of new symptom-formations ...

.... The doctrine of the universal neurosis of mankind, if we take it seriously, therefore compels us to entertain the hypothesis that the pattern of history exhibits a dialectic not hitherto recognized by historians, the dialectic of neurosis.[10]

Brown goes on to say "a reinterpretation of human history is not only an appendage to psychoanalysis but an integral part of it."[10] He emphasizes that "Freud not only maintains that human history can be understood only as a neurosis but also that the neuroses of individuals can be understood only in the context of human history as a whole."[10]

Whether we like Freud's views or not is irrelevant when it comes to the use of Freudian theories in interpreting historical developments. Freudian thought has had a tremendous impact on society and human behavior, and its influence is most relevant to historical research into the psychological makeup of women and men. There are numerous other psychologies we must draw on as well, namely the thinking of Carl Jung and Alfred Adler, humanistic psychology and the newly emerging field of transpersonal psychology.

The application of psychological theories in historical research has given rise to a whole new approach to the study of history, called psychohistory. Much has been written about this approach. Lifton explains its development:

Radical historical moments like ours—characterized by extraordinary intensity of change, inertia, and threat—call forth equally radical responses. This applies not only to social action but to modes of investigation as well. One example of what might be called investigative radicalism is the current intellectual effort ... to apply psychological methods to the study of historical patterns, present and past. This psychohistorical approach, however, is more than a mere expression of social upheaval. It stems from a general uneasiness among practitioners of both psychology and history about the capacity of their traditional methods to describe and explain man during the latter part of the twentieth century. And a specific uneasiness about certain conventional stances of their professions. . . .: The psychologist's tendency to eliminate history; and the historian's impulse to ignore, or else improvise poorly, psychological man.[11]

Lifton describes his own work in psychohistory as an effort to "explore ways in which men and women—some of them exposed to the most extreme experiences of our extreme epoch—suffer, survive, adapt, and evolve new modes of feeling and thought, of rebellion, and of life."[11] Lifton's work "suggest(s) systematic ways of studying and interpreting . . . diverse, and in some degree unprecedented, human developments."[11]

Nurses need to do research that will provide psychohistorical profiles of living nurses; we need to know their feelings, their thoughts and what has served to give meaning to their lives. This type of research can be of great benefit to future generations of nurses. Young practitioners entering the profession will be able to compare their own experiences with those of nurses who have gone before them, a comparison useful in preventing many of the struggles nurses have lived with in the past.

CREATIVE OPENNESS: FACING NEW HORIZONS IN RESEARCH

These suggestions for historical studies in nursing barely touch the surface of what needs to be done in this area of research. History opens wide opportunities for creative activity by nurses. Modern researchers recognize historical investigation as the parent of various sciences, including anthropology, archeology, biology, sociology, economics, political science, psychology and linguistics. Long before these offspring emerged as well-defined sciences, they were a part of historical investigation and writing. These sciences are still viewed as the "handmaidens" of the historian, who draws heavily from their bodies of knowledge and studies their development both as history made and as history in the making.[1]

The study of history gives people their identity and their philosophical reasons for being. For the sake of our own developing science and art within nursing, certain accepted assumptions about our role in society and its organizations must be questioned. Creative approaches to this questioning can generate exciting developments in nursing research and writing. Just as the foundation for scholarship in nursing should be creativity, this creativity should itself be founded on a reexamination of our history, an examination that will take us in our thinking well beyond the boundaries and limitations we have lived with in the past.

Scholars in various disciplines are becoming aware that research in the social sciences has not begun to solve our social and human problems. One critic argues that inquiry will increasingly be "turning inward toward the mechanisms of the knower's mind" or toward the study of "states of mind and their causes—states of mind such as happiness, bad temper and boredom."[12] He concludes that the traditional methods of experimental science do not lend themselves to the full and adequate exploration of human emotions.

In the cultivation of ourselves as artists and scientists, self-knowledge and self-understanding are of paramount importance. As we understand ourselves and our emotions more fully, we can feel more secure and more competent when working with both healthy clients and acutely ill ones. With creativity as our base, and with strong historical knowledge and awareness, nurses can become pioneers in developing new types of inquiry as inquiry itself shifts away from experimental science and turns inward toward self-knowledge and self-understanding.

REFERENCES

1. Barzun, J., & Graff, H. F. (1970). *The modern researcher* (pp. 54, 55, 176, 218). New York: Harcourt, Brace & World, Inc.

2. Arendt, H. (1958). *The human condition* (p. 190). Chicago: The University of Chicago Press.

3. May, R. (1975). *The courage to create* (pp. 59–60, 160). New York: W. W. Norton.

4. Williams, W. A. (1961). *The contours of American history* (p. 479). Chicago: Quadrangle Books.

5. May, R. (1972). *Power and innocence* (p. 56). New York: W. W. Norton & Co., Inc.

6. Tholfsen, T. R. (1967). *Historical thinking* (pp. 6–7). New York: Harper & Row.

7. Berlin, I. (1966). "The Concept of Scientific History." In W. H. Dray (Ed.), *Philosophical analysis and history* (pp. 40–41). New York: Harper & Row.

8. Williams, W. A. (1964). *The great evasion* (p. 18). Chicago: Quadrangle Books.

9. Marx, K., & Engels, F. (1974). *The communist manifesto* (pp. 57–58). New York: Washington Square Press.

10. Brown, N. O. (1959). *Life against death: The psychoanalytical meaning of history* (pp. 11–12). Middleton, CT: Wesleyan University Press.

11. Lifton, R. J. (1961). *History and human survival* (pp. 1–2, 12). New York: Random House, Vintage Books.

12. Hampshire, S. (1977, March 31). "The future of knowledge." *The New York Review of Books*, Vol. XXIV, No. 3 p. 14–18.

Building a Sound Foundation

Jo Ann Ashley

Building a solid foundation must
Grow out of careful thought,
Careful feeling, careful being.
This foundation must be built upon
Meaning in our own personal
    experience.

Experience is all that can give real
Meaning,
Be that experience one's own or the
Experience of another.
Experience is rooted in our being and
In our world of reality.

Building a foundation requires that
We express what we see as being real.
Our perceptions are of paramount
Importance.
These cannot be substituted for the
Perceptions of another.

If your experience agrees in
    substance
With mine,
If your perceptions of the world
    accord
With mine,

I can know from whence your thoughts
And feelings come.
Knowing this, I can decide if your
Journey and destination are the same
As mine.

Building a solid foundation takes
Strength that resides inside.
It will not do to always look outside.
Come share your dreams with me and
Together we can decide upon the
    design
Of the foundation we will fashion from
Our common experience, an
    experience
That dwells inside.

Outworn beliefs and lifestyles will
Not do as a basis for what we will
Build.
Dead theories and dirty politics
Cannot make our lives come alive.
To discard what is not meaningful
Is just what we must do.
My concern is eternity.
Is this your concern?

Chapter 12

MYTHS AND REALITIES OF APPRENTICESHIP IN NURSING

Paternalism in Practice*

INTRODUCTION: PURPOSE, PROBLEM, AND THEMES

*T*he purpose of historical research is primarily that of understanding the past, of providing an explanation of the forces shaping the development of an individual, a group, or a nation. Mere descriptive data or a chronologic recording of events and facts about people or institutions is useful as a limited source of information, but it is not necessarily good historical research or even truthful history.

Descriptive history is about the only kind which we have in nursing to date. Mostly based on nursing sources our history as written and published thus far can be called "house history." This kind of history does not shed light on continuity, diversity, and change, the very substance of historical research. With such limited historical research, we cannot hope to break the chains of the past or come to any clear understanding of where we have been, of where we are presently in our

---

* Paper presented at Teachers College, Columbia University, Thirteenth Annual Stewart Research Conference in Nursing, Friday, March 7, 1975.

development, or of where we should direct our energies for favorable change in the future.

A quote from William Appleman Williams further explains the purpose and value of historical research:

> History as a way of learning has one additional value beyond establishing the nature of reality and posing the questions that arise from its complexities and contradictions. It can offer examples of how other men faced up to the difficulties and opportunities of their eras. Even if the circumstances are noticeably different, it is illuminating, and productive of humility as well, to watch other men make their decisions, and to consider the consequences of their values and methods. If the issues are similar, then the experience is more directly valuable. But in either case the procedure can transform history as a way of learning into a way of breaking the chains of the past.[1]

In undertaking this research, it was my hope to at least identify more fully the chains of the past that bind nursing, if not to break them. The main purpose of this study was that of attempting to provide an explanation of why apprenticeship education survived so long in nursing when all other professional groups had largely moved away from this form of education shortly after the turn of the century. I raised the question, why did nursing have to contend with the problems growing out of apprenticeship when all other professions in America did not? I further concluded that paternalism or patriarchal views about women must have had a major impact on shaping nursing's development since nurses were women. Knowing that an accurate analysis of nursing's history could not be separated from a study of hospitals, I then raised specific research questions about apprenticeship, paternalism and how they were related to nursing's development in hospitals.

The year 1948 was selected as a cut-off point for the study since mid-century was near and the nursing profession was more than half a century old. By that time numerous official and unofficial studies of apprenticeship in nursing had been completed, the Goldmark Report of 1923 and the Brown Report of 1948 to name only two. Still, these studies and others did not provide any real or intellectually satisfying explanation of the survival of apprenticeship in a modern age. The reason for this lack of explanation was, I thought, the lack of any analysis of apprenticeship as a social phenomena. Also, paternalism as a factor influencing nursing and apprenticeship had been completely ignored, despite the obvious fact that nurses were women.

To comment briefly on the limitations of this research, like all dissertations mine is a scholarly piece of work limited in its provision of insightful interpretations. It is more descriptive than interpretative. For this reason, in the presentation of this paper, I wish to go a step beyond the dissertation sharing with you some of the results of my most recent reflections on the meaning of the data collected.

For almost five years now my thinking has been a bit fuzzy on this topic. As a researcher, I hasten to add, I do not feel badly about this "fuzziness" since the subject of my research is one that has puzzled nurses for a century and not one among us has dared to explore the problem, though it has had pervasive effects on women and on health care delivery in this country. In other words, the problems surrounding apprenticeship and paternalism in nursing are not ones easily explained in a dissertation or in a paper. And I do not expect to resolve your intellectual curiosity on the topic, but I do hope to arouse it.

The myths surrounding apprenticeship and paternalism in nursing gave rise to realities and practices not readily changed by the women who were early leaders in this profession. Even now, the myths they lived by are being examined by few scholars in nursing. The realities of our history have not been researched and analyzed to an extent sufficient for understanding these myths and the social order shaping the formation of modern nursing. Nurses still live and cope with the myths, realities and practices, the roots of which became established in the nineteenth and early part of the twentieth century. These are the themes of this paper. The chains of our past are the damaging effects suffered by nursing throughout its history as a result of abuses growing out of social attitudes about women. Nursing's growth was shaped by these attitudes and by the social context of the times.

THE SOCIAL CONTEXT

Hospital Development in America: Business versus
Humanitarian and Charitable Motivations

First, I will comment briefly on the social context influencing developments in the health care system. In America, the growth of hospitals was primarily a manifestation of the charitable instinct motivating public-spirited individuals to provide care for the indigent sick, who at a time of illness and dependency, could not help themselves. Rather than looking solely to their government for providing care to the sick poor, private individuals set out to devise a means of helping the poorer working-class citizens regain health and thus remain useful to themselves and the community. Almshouses, a system of poor relief, existed to house the destitute and homeless, but a stigma was attached to these institutions; people entered them, not for help, but to die or receive food and shelter. They were not institutions providing medical and nursing care.

A Philadelphia physician conceived the idea of establishing an institution solely for the purpose of treatment and nursing care of the sick, in or about the year 1750. This physician consulted with Benjamin Franklin on the "business end" of the "beneficent design." It was Benjamin Franklin who wrote the petition for establishing the first American Hospital.

Presented to the Pennsylvania Assembly in 1751, Franklin's petition proposed the founding of an institution "novel" to Americans. The purpose of this institution was to provide nursing treatment for individuals having homes, but lacking the means to obtain nursing and medical treatment when burdened with a disease rendering them unable to continue providing for themselves and their families. A clear distinction was made between the hospital and the almshouse, the latter for poor relief, was seen as an unfit place to recover from illness.

Not financed by public monies, this first American hospital was then a semi-private corporation, supported by private subscriptions and paying patients. Those sponsoring its development felt they could provide a necessary service both better than and different from that provided the poor through governmental support. The first hospital did accept those totally unable to pay, but of necessity, one of the earliest sources of revenue came from patients who could and were required to pay.

Although an outgrowth of charitable impulse, the actual incorporation and operation of America's first hospitals were influenced by no less of a business mind than that of Benjamin Franklin's. Hospital care in America began neither as a system of poor relief nor as a free service. To Benjamin Franklin health services offered to the working poor were "privileges," not rights. Those who could pay should pay and did pay.

The main point I wish to make is that although associated with charitable activities, hospitals have never been charitable institutions in the strict sense of the word. Both public and private hospitals have always accepted paying and non-paying patients. But, for the sake of reputation, private hospitals have accepted the poor also, keeping their numbers to a minimum. Hospital care is big business and hospitals today have less of a charitable and humanistic inclination than at any previous point in our history.

Significantly, prior to Florence Nightingale, hospitals were unsafe places for patients. People went there to die, not to get well. Most people, with the exception of the homeless, were reluctant to enter hospitals. The development of modern nursing and the application of scientific knowledge by nurses was the factor leading to the transformation of hospitals in both England and America. Not until the profession of nursing became a reality did these institutions have a service to offer the sick that made them well. We have all heard, read, and been told that the medical profession deserves credit for the transformation of hospitals, but this is a myth, not based on fact. Created by propaganda dispensed by medicine and reinforced by sociological studies not based on sound historical research, this myth has added to the prestige of the medical profession and perpetuated misconceptions about nursing.

The increasing interest of the medical profession in hospitals was the major factor prompting hospital authorities to view their problems from more of a business efficiency rather than a humanitarian stand-point. The tendency of physicians to think along business lines is reflected in much of the early writings appearing in medical journals.

The development of a business ideology along with professionalization on the part of the medical profession had numerous effects on hospitals. In the first place, physicians' ideas were significant because many held executive positions in the hospital field and determined policies. Secondly, medical men eventually came to use the hospital in some capacity while at the same time remaining in the position of independent entrepreneurs, not responsible for the operating costs of these institutions.

The medical profession's belief in the economic philosophy of individualism and their efforts to maintain laissez faire approaches in health care accounts for the development of hospitals as businesses in this country. Despite their growth as businesses, hospitals managed to maintain what I have called a charitable mystique. Their association with charitable endeavors has persisted when in reality their operation has been influenced more by a business ideology and economic considerations than by humanitarian and charitable motives.

The charitable mystique, a myth widely accepted by nurses and the public, had profound effects on the survival of apprenticeship education in nursing. The system of private enterprise in the health field provided ideal circumstances for giving rise to the creation of oppressive conditions for women. Women did not cope well with conditions in a capitalistic society serving to oppress them. The trend toward establishing apprenticeship programs, not as independent educational enterprises, but as business arrangements to supply a source of subordinate labor managed by hospitals, is illustrated by the manner in which the growth of programs paralleled that of hospitals. In one decade alone, 1900 to 1910, well over a thousand new hospitals were established, many were small, private, profit-making institutions. This was an era of unprecedented growth both for apprentice programs for women and for institutions caring for the sick. Also, by 1910, there were well over a thousand schools.

The influence of a business ideology in a growing hospital industry was incentive enough for the exploitation of women's labor. The apprenticeship system provided an ideal structure and a socially acceptable means for the exploitation of large numbers of women. Because of the myth that hospitals were charitable institutions doing only good for the sick in society, the public accepted the practice of exploiting women while hospitals promised them education. In reality, the vast majority of apprentice programs established prior to the 1930s and 1940s were not schools at all, but a means of supplying cheap labor. This climate and the supporting social attitudes about women presented severe impediments to nursing's development.

The Status of Women

Prior to 1900, apprenticeship was the acceptable route into numerous professions, not just nursing. Early nurses, like all women, had to contend with a very low social status. In nursing, formal programs were an outgrowth of the efforts of women to provide proof of their social and economic worth outside of the home, and their success in doing so was an innovative experiment in the field of women's education. Financed by the payment of one's education with one's labor, apprenticeship was a cheap plan requiring no public support from a monetary standpoint. The American public readily embraced it as an acceptable form of education for women, since it did not involve their movement into institutions of higher education. Of paramount importance to both hospitals and communities, it served a utilitarian function of obvious value to the public.

At the time apprenticeship for women was publicly accepted, nineteenth century Victorian ideas persisted and the intellectual development of women was thought to be harmful to their actual physical growth and normal functioning. Women did not, of course, have any political status, not even the right to vote. Socially, they had moved forward because of their involvement in the humanitarian movements of the nineteenth century. Their accomplishments had been recognized as a social good and a social necessity, but this visibility did not result in their obtaining political freedom or a legal status. The low status of women was a factor having a significant impact on the nursing profession from the beginning of its inception.

By 1900, nurses were clearly the equals of physicians in their training and in their contributions to the health care of society. However, they were not their equals in the political and economic spheres of human activity and influence in the society, and it was their lack of equality in the latter that would shape their development far more than their professional potential and aspirations. It was economic, political, and derivative social factors that impeded progress, keeping their contributions and reforms of apprenticeship to a minimum until mid-century. It is still these factors that keep the contributions of nurses in health care low.

At the very outset, early leaders in nursing were less than attuned to the ramifications of the problems women faced in a society where they had no political freedom, no legal status, and literally no rights to become professional persons. They were lacking in a full appreciation of the extent to which social inequality with men would be used against them, preventing them from modifying their status for nearly a century. As second-class citizens, the myths and prejudices directed toward women for centuries were destined to influence the for-formation and growth of American nursing, leading to the survival of apprenticeship and the institutionalization of paternalism.

REALITIES OF APPRENTICESHIP IN NURSING

The most significant finding of my research is that decade after decade few changes were accomplished in bringing about improvements in nursing education and practice. The flexibility and lack of planning characteristic of laissez faire approaches allowed hospitals to do as they pleased with no outside authorities-ties to evaluate standards and practices employed. Hospitals could grow, and did grow as businesses, but the consequences for the growth of a woman's profession was something else again. No laissez faire atmosphere surrounded or modified the myths about women; these were rigid and inflexible. Nursing, after 1910, entered a period of stagnation, lasting forty years with few innovations.

Partly to illustrate the historical roots of some of nursing problems and to delineate the major influences, impeding its social and professional development, I want to comment upon some of the concerns of early leaders in nursing. These concerns can be classified into three major categories. First, of primary concern was that of improving standards. It was their hope and professional aspiration to establish uniform standards that would be universally accepted in all hospital schools. A second concern was that of changing the public concept of nursing as an activity performed by amateurs or untrained women into one of a practice engaged in by professionally trained and knowledgeable women who could be socially productive, receiving economic rewards for their efforts, a goal sought after by all professional groups. Finally, leaders were concerned about the lack of legal status of nurses and the problems this created in regulating those who engaged in practice.

The Problem of Standards

In regard to the first category of concerns regarding standards, leaders could not accomplish this goal because the hospital schools were privately owned and each individual hospital decided what standards they would or would not observe. Officials repeatedly argued that the numbers of students and the standards should be determined by the needs of the hospital for service and by the economic laws of supply and demand. Hospitals set the hours of labor for students and determined what courses would or would not be taught in their schools. Hospitals operated their apprentice programs with no regard for the standards recommended by organized nursing. Only the most reputable hospitals even considered these recommendations as worthy of any notice, whether they implemented proposed changes or not. Exploitation was rampant, accepted with little questioning by the women who entered the programs or by the larger society.

As a result of the private ownership of schools, proposals for improve-improvements made by organized nursing in the 1890s did not become a reality in the majority of schools until 1950. One example should be sufficient to illustrate the slowness of change: the concept of affiliation, though proposed as early as 1888, did not become a common feature in the majority of schools until the 1950s. Affiliation between hospitals for educational purposes was opposed for both economic and psychological reasons. Hospital officials argued that students could not be spared from the service role in the home hospital and many expressed the fear that students on affiliation might lose their feelings of loyalty to the home hospital.

The American Hospital Association and the American Medical Association were active opponents to all elevations of standards and their organized opposition began in the first decade of the century. Instead of seriously (or I should say openly and publicly), questioning this opposition, leaders in nursing sought approval of physicians and they became active participants in the activities of the American Hospital Association.

Initial efforts of nurses to cooperate with the hospital association actually began in 1908 and 1909 with the formation of the latter's committee on training schools. As committeewomen, leaders in nursing gave their input to that association's organized efforts to intensify its control over the schools and the standards which should or should not be implemented. Their participation as committeewomen very shortly led to their absorption into the hospital association. Within the second decade of the century, members of the National League for Nursing actually joined forces with their oppressors by becoming associate members of the hospital association. At this level of membership, the women had no voting power and no influence on the policies of the American Hospital Association, although many faithfully attended meetings to present their problems.

This behavior on the part of nursing leaders was damaging to the efforts of their own professional organizations. By supporting the hospital association and by seeking this organization's approval for reforms, they actually negated their own professional goals. Policy makers in the American Hospital Association were not concerned about the education of the nurse since hospital schools were really business arrangements serving the purposes of management very well. Time and again hospital officials admitted to leaders that they (the hospital administration) made profits off of nursing schools. Instead of putting this money into the development of the schools and innovations in nursing practice, or even the employment of hospital graduates to staff hospitals, profits made off of student nurses were put into the development of other hospital departments, though nursing care was the major service provided by these institutions. This was an economic abuse blatantly unfair to women and damaging to the nursing profession and quality care.

While male-dominated groups within the health field made progress, women in nursing did not and could not under the repressive circumstances surrounding the operation of apprenticeship. And because the larger society also discriminated against nurses, the profession was bound to the apprenticeship system and the hospital. Colleges and universities assumed little responsibility for this field of women's education. Nursing leaders had, from 1911 on, attempted to establish connections with institutions of higher education, but here failure was built into their efforts. Until recently, the connections they did establish with these institutions were scarcely better than the arrangements they already had with hospitals. Throughout nursing's history, educational problems derived from the economic abuse of women along with the social discrimination preventing the intellectual development of nurses, all an outgrowth of sexual prejudice. Standards remained low, preventing progress in improving quality health care for citizens.

Domestic Servants versus Professional Practitioners

In regard to the second category of concerns, changing the public concept of nursing as an activity engaged in by professionals as opposed to amateurs, here again economic considerations and prejudice prevented the realization of this goal. And nurses are still trying to convince the public that they are professionals. This issue has never been resolved largely because society has denied women the rights of becoming recognized professionals, with expertise equal to men.

The very structural complexity of nursing, with all of its levels, grew out of the controversy over the untrained versus the professionally trained nurse engaging in practice for compensation. Historically, the origins of levels in nursing had nothing to do with distinctions between technical and professional practice. On the basis of my research findings, this current explanation of the levels in an attempt to rationalize what in fact is a phenomena resulting from the economic abuses directed toward the nursing profession, abuses demeaning to women and their right to be professionals with the privilege of being free from unfair competition.

The main factor giving rise to levels within nursing was that physicians, hospitals, and commercial groups, and even some nurses, all argued that any woman regardless of educational background should be allowed to practice nursing for the economic rewards to be obtained in an open market. Thus, both the untrained and partially trained women all entered nursing, and were encouraged to do so in large numbers. Many came from short courses established by physicians, ranging from six weeks to two months; this was a popular route into nursing. These workers were called "sub-nurses" and were the forerunners of practical nurses, and the present technical nurse.

This development was really an outgrowth of social injustices and inequality for both women and the lower classes in society, since it was argued that sub-nurses could give care to the poor who did not deserve better care by the better prepared nurses. Physicians sponsoring the cause of sub-nurses firmly believed that nursing was nothing more than domestic service which all women could engage in; they also believed that the poor deserved a lesser quality of nursing care than did the wealthy.

Hospital graduates were considered a "luxury" that society could not afford. The sub-nurses knew little or nothing about symptoms, disease, or nursing treatment and the sick who employed their services received no nursing care. Given the predominance of private enterprise in health care, nursing was dispensed in an open market with no controls on prices or on standards to regulate those who practiced as nurses. Thus, families might well end up with "housekeepers of the sick" while paying for the services of what they thought to be the fully trained, not knowing the difference. This practice was sanctioned by the law and by reputable physicians, as well as hospitals and commercial employment agencies.

Failure to have nursing recognized as a service equal in professional value to services provided by professions dominated by men grew out of myths that women should be wives and mothers, not professional persons making a social contribution and sharing equally with men in the economic life of the society. Both social and economic abuses derived from these myths and resulting realities in practice. Unemployment among nurses was a constant problem along with the gross exploitation of the public. In addition to the unfair competition, subnurses also served to keep the public image of nursing low, as indicated by survey in the 1930s and 1940s. Conditions of employment were so poor many women refused to enter the field while others left to live by the myths urging them to be wives and mothers.

Legalized Inequality and Subservience

Status problems have survived, largely because nurses are women. The political power of organized nursing was less than effective in bringing about real social reforms; more powerful groups in the health field did not want reforms and continued to actively oppose them. This brings me to a discussion of the third category of concerns, the legal status of nurses.

The registration movement to aid legal status began in the first decade of the century. Nurses had identified and organized themselves as professionals and wanted the societal sanctions and protections readily accorded other groups. Since nursing along with medicine and dentistry was one of the three earliest professions organized in the health field, nurses wanted legal recognition like that obtained by dentists and doctors. This was reasonable enough, but since nurses were women without political freedom or a legal status, they were second-class citizens and with the enactment of the early nurse practice acts they were destined to become second-class professionals as well.

Nurses did obtain legal recognition through their efforts. This recognition did not, however provide them with political, economic, or professional freedom. Instead, enactment of the early laws only made more evident the subservient role of nurses as women who did not have the right to become professionals, independent of male-dominated groups.

Early registration laws only gave public sanction to the already existing condition of the subjection of nurses to physicians. The laws merely recognized the state of inequality between men and women in the health field, they did not correct them. At the same time legalized inequality became a reality, granting men the right to dominate women, the laws did not protect nurses or the public from abuses fostered by the development of sub-nurses. In effect, the laws granted few privileges and no legal protection to nurses or the public. We have not yet corrected legalized inequality between men and women in the health field, this movement has only begun. Thus, historically, the laws of the land repressed nurses quite as effectively as the system of apprenticeship did with its economic abuses.

BINDING MYTHS: PATERNALISM IN PRACTICE

Already bound to hospitals through apprenticeship with its restrictions and impediments to growth, the early laws bound nurses to the authority of physicians. Not only did the early nurses have their professional rights and privileges negated, the laws perpetuated the social concept that nursing was not a profession requiring any degree of expertise and knowledge, but a domestic service to be engaged in by any woman. The myth that women should remain subservient to men was legalized and with that, paternalism in practice was institutionalized. Men and women alike live by myths which order and give meaning to the roles they play. Myths and accompanying realities influencing nursing's development were grossly discriminatory to women in the field and should have been more seriously examined and destroyed long ago. For as the times change, our myths should also change. Those no longer useful in achieving healthy development should be discarded and new ones created. The chains of the past can be broken, and new learning and new roles become a reality only through the process of understanding and modifying unhealthy myths having harmful effects on the social and economic order of a society and upon the lives of individuals whose actions shape the future for all people.

Mythological symbols in nursing blinded young women to the truth of realities in practice. Our use of white as a symbol representing purity, innocence, and dignity were deceptive. While nurses were taught that they belonged to "an honorable profession," the whole of society would not accord them this status, or provide the conditions and support needed to enable them to understand the deception in myths that bound them to roles in which they were not free to be professionals, with privileges equal to men. The symbols of white cap, shoes, and dress attracted women into nursing, but such symbols illustrate the manner in which myths can become deceptive and oppressive without constant examination and modification. Our oppressive symbols have not been analyzed from a historical point of view and we know few of the truths about our roots. Walking many miles in our white shoes, we were cast in the role of beasts of burden, or at the least, as sheep, unaware that we were being deceived. The lamps we supposedly carried did not light our way to insight, nor did the oath we took guide us to truth and what was for us a right as professionals.

Under the guise of charitable activity, hospitals perpetuated the evils apprenticeship and nurses along with the public believed, for a century, that these institutions were doing good when in fact they were doing harm to both. Nurses have not been alone in their deception for the public too has not known the extent to which our myths have bound us to the past in the health care system, resulting in poor quality care.

Another myth serving to restrict nurses has been the "godlike status" assumed by physicians. Some nurses have always known that physicians, underneath their thin veil of authority and superiority, were not "gods," but ordinary men committing errors, just like nurses and other mortal men. Nurses have not questioned this myth to any extent, and its effects upon them. Its harmful influences on nursing and health care should receive more research emphasis in the future.

IMPLICATIONS FOR FUTURE RESEARCH

Nurses have walked in the shadow of physicians and hospital administrators, not aware that this very position blocked their vision and public visibility, preventing their growth as professionals. It is now time to unmask the veiled history of both nursing and medicine. For too long now all of us—educators, practitioners, and researchers—have avoided raising questions about and investigating the truths that lie hidden within our history. I have primarily discussed the negative aspects of myths that have bound us to a lack of progress. Contemporary nurses have, I believe, internalized the collective burden of guilt resulting from social injustices heaped upon our profession and women. We need research that can help us externalize this guilt for it belongs to the whole of society more than to us, though we are not totally without blame since our leaders in practice and teachers have not seriously sought to understand our history. Out of ignorance of the past, nurses themselves have strengthened the chains binding them with no thought of analyzing the nature of these.

We are at a point in our historical development where, in many instances, so-called innovations are not innovations but a repeating of past errors under the guise of change and progress. To date our research, for the most part, is shallow, lacking in meaningful insights about nurses themselves or about the true nature of nursing phenomena. Often through our research efforts, we create little knowledge that can be shared with other disciplines or little knowledge that can be used by future generations in their attempts to create a new and better world, a world without prejudice that stifles human growth, health, and creativity.

By not concentrating serious research attention on the ramifications of social, psychological, and economic problems faced by women in nursing, our behavior has been somewhat like that of a dog, an underdog at that, chasing its tail, going around in circles, constantly on the move but getting nowhere. Real change if it is to become a reality in practice will of necessity require this type of basic and meaningful research. Unsure of our own historical base of knowledge, we have operated out of a sense of insecurity having the tendency to believe and accept without question research that has perpetuated myths and misconceptions about us.

Very often, the designs and methods of collecting data on nursing phenomena do not make a good fit when applied to nursing. Like wearing clothes not designed for our size and weight, they fit us too tightly or too loosely and we look poorly as a result. We need to know more about the history of practice in nursing in order to develop designs that fit our phenomena and with which we can be more comfortable. We need new and fresh approaches in research derived from a study of the unexplored mysteries surrounding the myths and realities which have shaped us into who we are today. There is a positive as well as a negative side to myths and it is the positive side that we must learn more about to guide our growth in the future.

REFERENCE

1. Williams, W. A. (1961). *The contours of American history* (p. 479). Chicago: Quadrangle Books.
2. Ashley, J. A. (1972). *Hospital sponsorship of nursing schools: Influence of apprenticeship and paternalism on nursing education in America, 1893–1948.* (Doctoral dissertation, Teachers College, Columbia University. Publication as *Nurse work: Medical paternalism and American health care* (Summer, 1975). New York: Teachers College Press.

PART FOUR

NEW HORIZONS FOR
NEW NURSES

*T*he rites of passage that celebrate the transition from student to graduate can provide contrasting views on nursing. In these last two papers, Dr. Ashley addresses the ceremonies of academic commencement and the tradition of the nursing pinning ceremony. Today these ceremonies often coexist in an uneasy tension between the traditions of hospital-based nursing that long predominated and nursing's move into the realm of university education. The focus on academic achievement in collegiate education and loyalty and obedience in diploma nursing education highlights the competing world views on the education of women in this century. As Dr. Ashley observes, ceremonies embody powerful myths and symbols that give meaning to our professional and personal lives.

Patriarchy and paternalism have persisted as a means of social control through much of nursing's history. Long viewed as women's work, nursing has been torn apart by the struggle to gain access to higher education and to develop as a respected academic discipline. Initially, sexism in higher education assisted the system of diploma education to grow by barring women from entrance to colleges and education. As nursing evolved under a system of apprenticeship, in the hospital institution it became devalued. Nurses were handmaidens to the physician, and their education was rooted in implementing skills, not ideas. Despite the intellectual brilliance of nursing founders such as Florence Nightingale, Adelaide Nutting, and Isabel Hampton Robb, nursing adapted to the growing pursuit of scientific management. Viewed also as manual labor, the pursuit of an intellectual basis for nursing practice was discouraged not only by medicine and hospital administrators, but also by many nurses.

As Ashley points out, the prestige of the ideology and the dominance it exerted was so great that many nurses embraced the altruistic notion of service and rejected the pursuit of higher education. This anti-intellectualism marginalized the perceived threat that nursing autonomy and professionalism posed. Also, many women found the conditions of diploma nursing education and hospital service more tolerable than in the mills or as domestic servant. Nursing education reinforced the conception of ideal womanhood, training women not only in patient care, but in a social demeanor of docility and subordination to medicine. Mythology about nursing continued to reflect the patriarchal expectations of the "good woman." For example, nurses were told:

- "It takes a good woman to make a good nurse."
- "Nursing is good preparation for marriage and children."
- "A good nurse is born and not made."
- "Nursing is a good career to fall back on . . . you can always get a job and . . ."

This anti-intellectualism persists today, with nurses often confronted with the adage "you are much too bright to be a nurse, why didn't you become a doctor?" As Ashley observes, old but powerful ideas about the nature of womanhood and nursing have bound and still bind and limit nursing potential.

The two papers in this section capture Dr. Ashley's concern for the future of nursing. As a historian, she recorded distance traveled by nursing on its path to autonomous professionalism, but lamented the persistence of patriarchy blocking the journey. As an educator, she was keenly aware of the pull that graduates perceive between the idealism of education and the reality of practice. Her belief in the human potential for change through social activism compelled her to go beyond her critical perspective to offer hope and encouragement for nursing. She was committed to the liberation of nurses. The power of her words were directed to opening the eyes and freeing the minds of nurses, so that they could shed their outdated myths and symbols.

Breaking away from old boundaries and limitations is the central theme of Dr. Ashley's paper addressed to the graduates of the 1977 School of Nursing at the University of Oregon Health Sciences Center. As in her other commencement addresses, Dr. Ashley urges graduates to use their power to break away from the boundaries and limitations inherent in narrow perspectives on nursing and to develop their intellectual and political potential. She saw the development of nursing theory as empowering and political savvy as a means to liberate nursing and benefit the public.

Dr. Ashley envisioned the use of nursing creativity as *the* force to set nursing free from the long-held view of "nursing['s] subordination to medicine." This relationship has hindered nurses from fully offering their care to the public. In the film documentary, *Nursing: The Politics of Caring* (Fanlight Films, 1978), Dr. Ashley spoke of the public's need for nursing care, nursing's ability to help people learn to care for themselves. An advocate for nursing clinics, or nursing centers of care for the public, she worked with her nursing students in the community to find creative models of nursing care. These experiences made her keenly aware of nursing's perceived threats to medicine and the political-legal barriers to her and similar efforts. Despite her own experiences, she was steadfast in her belief that nursing could circumvent the barriers and claim "a place in the sun."

As we approach the next century, new models of nursing practice are emerging across the country. Nursing centers funded by federal project monies continue to struggle for legitimacy and reimbursement, but have demonstrated their worth to the community. The nurse practitioner movement, while it has made major gains on a state-by-state basis, continues to confront barriers to practice and limitations on prescription writing and reimbursement. Despite ample research on the effectiveness of nursing care, there is a reluctance to legitimate nursing in the policy arena. Basic changes such as Medicare reimbursement of nurse practitioners or untying the provision of home care by nurses from the control of physicians are regretfully slow in occurring. Dr. Ashley expressed the concern that new models of care and new roles like the nurse practitioner's could not easily escape the prevailing effects of paternalism and patriarchy in healthcare. Her hope was that, in their new roles and models, nurses would reflect on their history and avoid repeating the mistakes of previous generations.

The final paper in this collection, "Reflections on Myths and Symbols Pinning Nursing Down," calls for unmasking the symbols and myths inherent in nursing culture. Dr. Ashley explores the traditions of the pinning ceremony. Noting that pinning entails "holding fast" or to keep within certain bounds, she suggests that the persistence of the pinning ceremony at a university school of nursing presents an irony. Together with lamps, caps, and white uniforms, the "nursing pin stands as a symbol of outdated mythology." Suggesting conformance with rules that were rooted in nineteenth-century attitudes of womanhood, religious values, and oppressive social life, Dr. Ashley acknowledged the value of myths and symbols to give meaning to human life. She cautions young graduates to look critically to make certain that their symbols do not oppress and stifle their growth and productivity.

Twenty years ago when Dr. Ashley wrote this paper, nurses were being fired for not wearing their nursing caps. Today nurses may be found wearing street clothes and a variety of different colors of uniforms, and caps are viewed as a potential source of infectious diseases. Yet, the culture of pinning persists, with all types of nursing programs still conveying the pin as a symbol of the passage from student to nurse. The ambivalence of nursing educators in this regard, who struggled through the decades of the 1960s and 1970s, is confusing to young graduates. After striving to be identified as professionals and fighting for the right not to be ensconced in uniforms and rituals, the ritual of pinning reopens the wounds of painful struggles. Always sensitive to language, Ashley presents a wordplay and suggests that pinning be a "right of passage." In her poem, *If You Must Be Pinned*, she warns graduates away from the traditions of conformity, saying, "Let pinning be for you a symbol for defining your own boundaries, limits, and grooves." Dr. Ashley reminds us that the potential for nursing liberation from the myths and symbols of the past can be actualized through critical thought and action. Pinned together, the collective power and creativity of nurses would be a formidable force by which to revolutionize healthcare.

Chapter 13

THE EMERGENCE OF NEW HORIZONS IN NURSING

*A Timely Commencement**

BREAKING AWAY FROM OLD BOUNDARIES AND LIMITATIONS: EXPANDING HORIZONS

*A*s persons, each and every one of you, were born to live out your life in a period of social unrest. We live in a time of turmoil and uncertainty. Much of this turmoil and uncertainty can be found in the hearts and minds of human beings, and in the malfunctioning of our social institutions. From the standpoint of history, massive social unrest is an indicator of forthcoming change; and, the making of world shaking social change is surely in process. At the present time, the horizons of this change are not really visible because on many, many frontiers of knowledge expanding horizons are quite boundless and open with no well-defined conceptions of what the future of humanity may be like for living persons.

Currently, we have numerous reasons for being concerned about the changes we are undergoing in our society. It can be well-documented

---

* A commencement address at the graduation ceremony, class of 1977, School of Nursing, University of Orgeon Health Sciences Center, Portland, Oregon, June 11, 1977.

that we humans are becoming more and more aware of the fact that "boredom is increasingly the disease of advanced industrial civilization."[1] In an article about "The Future of Knowledge," Stuart Hampshire describes this ailment as a pervasive "sense of triviality, a sense that one is a replaceable part in a mechanism, in no way distinct and indispensable."[2] Still others describe this ailment as a sense of "lostness" and comment upon our being witness to the era of "man as robot" or "man as machine." Our modern condition has been described as "an unforgettable portrait of modern man and woman in the process of losing their person and their humanity."[3]

Some critics of modern industrial society firmly believe our society will crumble and fall like ancient Rome. Still others maintain a more optimistic view believing our age is an age of both disintegration and reintegration, an age giving rise to the development of new values and new institutions.

This phenomena of disintegration and reintegration is described by Stavrianos eminent world historian in his book entitled *The Promise of the Coming Dark Age*. This historian notes that the "circumstances of the fall of Rome and the advent of the Dark Ages are very relevant to the present world."[4] According to this researcher, the similarities between our own time and Roman times are the following: "(1) economic imperialism, (2) ecological degradation, (3) bureaucratic ossification, and (4) a flight from reason."[5]

In one form or another, all of these phenomena are evident in today's world. As this relates to your own personal future, you will be working in a system grossly affected by these phenomena. In the American health care system, economic imperialism, bureaucratic ossification, and a flight from reason are basic features of this system. Manifestations of these are reflected in the numerous problems we can observe in the health field; not the least of these problems is the personal degradation of workers and the gross dehumanization of patients.

Presenting these bleak-sounding interpretations about developments in our society does not mean that we cannot, in our thinking, capitalize on more optimistic interpretations having much brighter overtones. For example, clear and distinct movements are underway in society, movements led by people who are no longer willing to accept the blatant negation of their precious humanity. These people may well be taking action to overcome their sense of boredom, but the actions themselves are resulting in changed values and changed perceptions of the world on the part of many persons. Since all of you were born to live in a period of social unrest such as ours, you can rejoice and be exceedingly glad about these movements. These movements are giving rise to the emergence of new horizons in nursing and in the realm of knowledge itself.

As you know quite well, you have been educated to enter a woman's profession. Therefore, one movement I want to focus attention on is the feminist movement. Women are beginning to realize that dead and dying theories about the nature of human behavior fall far short of saying much that is meaningful about the true nature of woman. Theories and conceptual frameworks growing out of patriarchal ideations have been damaging to women's health, their self-image, and their sense of well-being. Women, as a result of this damage, are finally awakening from a sound sleep and are beginning to question theories in fields ranging from religion to economics and politics. Although women are not likely to advocate the development of a matriarchal social order, they, at the same time, want to shed the burden of carrying the heavy weight of the patriarchal cross for a much longer period of time. For health reasons alone, women must develop their powers of thought and action in different directions. Liberated women want to freely use their own minds to develop their own theories to explain the realities of the world and to shape ideals related to conceptions of what that world ought to be like.

With the questioning of theories, much information that has been accepted as factual is in the process of being reordered, revised, and updated to accord with the experiences of living persons. The mutability of knowledge is a well-known fact that does not change. Science itself must alter and modify "its interpretations every few years, and on its frontiers hypotheses conflict."[6] The development of women as theorists, as scientists, and as artists will inevitably bring with it vast changes in our thought processes and in our perceptions of the world we live in. Emerging from the depths of women's minds and beings, future horizons of thought about human behavior will look far different from what we have accepted as truth in the past.

Our theories of the future will present us with a more total view of related events than theories of the past have been able to present. I say this because in our patriarchal societies men have been the predominant generators and carriers of ideas; and, men in their development of theories and ideas to explain events in the world have been more biased than even they would care to openly admit.

Men have not only given birth to ideas, they have used these ideas to give shape and form to our values, our beliefs, and our social organizations. Our legal, economic, and political systems have also derived from these biased ideas. The boundaries and limitations placed upon women in these systems is precisely the focus of the feminist movement and they are perhaps the prime motive forces prompting women to seek new knowledge and new interpretations about human behavior and the functioning of society.

You are graduating at a time when human institutions are manifesting severe weaknesses and limitations in the extent to which they are able to solve social and human problems. In her book *The Human Condition*, Hannah Arendt comments upon the limitations of human institutions:

> Limitations and boundaries exist within the realm of human affairs, but they never offer a framework that can reliably withstand the onslaught with which each new generation must insert itself. The frailty of human institutions and laws and, generally, of all matters pertaining to men's living together, arises from the human condition of mortality and is quite independent of the frailty of human nature . . . the territorial boundaries which protect and make possible the physical identify of a people, and the laws which protect and make possible its political existence, are of such great importance to the stability of human affairs precisely because no such limiting and protecting principles rise out of the activities going on in the realm of human affairs itself. The limitations of the law are never entirely reliable safeguards against action from without. The boundlessness of action is only the other side of its tremendous capacity

for establishing relationships, that is, its specific productivity; this is why the old virtue of moderation, of keeping within bounds, is indeed one of the political virtues par excellence . . . [7]

Hannah Arendt is making some very important observations about human behavior and social institutions. She emphasizes that limitations and boundaries are not useful frameworks when social change is in order. This observation is fascinating when applied to women's role in society and especially when applied to the role of the nursing profession. Where nursing is concerned, a framework of limitations and boundaries has been *the* conceptual framework guiding our development for over a century. This conceptual approach has defined our professional identity, our political existence, and our relationships of power or powerlessness in the world of work. Our specific productivity in various economic and social organizations derive from boundaries and limitations very often not defined by our own aspirations, experiences, and cultivation of our ideas and our persons.

NARROW CONCEPTUAL VIEWS OF NURSES: OVERCOMING OBSTACLES TO GROWTH

Because of the boundaries and limitations placed upon us nurses, our perceptions of our place in health care, in society, and in the world have been narrow and limited. The time has come for individuals like you and like me to change these perceptions. To illustrate the nature of some of the limitations we have lived with, let me tell you a couple of true stories. Sometime ago, I spoke to a group of nurses in the state of Utah. At that meeting, a physician was also on the program of speakers. I spoke on the myths surrounding the commonly held view that nurses and medical doctors make an effective team in delivering health care to society.

After I presented my paper, the physician proceeded to present his views about physicians and nurses making a team. This physician compared the nurse-doctor team to a football team. He explained that on this team the physician was both coach and captain. In his perception of this team, we nurses were mere backup, supportive players and could have no role at all in deciding upon team strategies or plays to be made. Our role was perceived as a powerless one, narrow and limited. All we were supposed to do was to follow the leader with no intelligent forethought or insightful attention given to our actions related to patient care. The physician was the one to make all the decisions.

At the time, I informed this physician that I saw no comparison between a football team and a health care team. Though it determined this physician's perceptual views of the boundaries and limitations of the nurses' role, this comparison held no meaning for me. I do believe in liberating women to be whatever they want to be, even if this happens to be football players, but in any serious consideration of a health care team, I just had never imagined myself or nurses functioning in a capacity similar to that of football players. Where the welfare of society is concerned, our role is certainly not one of entertainment or amusement.

In describing his perceptions of the nurse's behavior, this physician went further to explain that the health care team was like a team of horses; as he explained it, every gang of horses has a leader that emerges and the rest of the horses follow where this leading horse leads them. At this point in our discussion, I told this physician I was born in Kentucky and knew quite well the difference between women and horses. Again, I saw absolutely no comparison between the health care team and a team of horses.

Needless to say, the mentality of this physician was appalling to me, but since that meeting in Utah I have come to understand the fact that physicians in no way consider the nurse their equal. Just recently in the state of Illinois, I was interviewed by a newspaper reporter. When the results of that interview were published, I was quoted as saying the nurse is equally as important as the physician in the delivery of quality care. After the publication of that true statement, grown men wearing the label of M.D. began to harass and threaten young student nurses with their comments and arguments that in no way could the nurse be the equal of the physician in value or in importance. Weeks after that newspaper article was published, these same physicians were still harassing my students and verbally attacking them for a comment I had made. These medical doctors have no concept of educated women like yourselves ever being their equal.

I have used these particular examples to illustrate a major point: across this country the vast majority of physicians and large segments of the public hold these same conceptual views of the nurse and her role as this relates to physicians and others in the health care field. For over a century now, these views of nurses and the nursing profession have set limits on our growth and expansion; these views of us have confined our functioning within narrow boundaries preventing us from delivering quality nursing and health care to a public which needs this care so badly.

A framework of boundaries and limitations is precisely what this generation of nurses—your generation, my generation—must break away from if we are to change the political, economic, and social systems in which we work, freeing us to do our work of nursing. We must break away from outdated conceptual views of the nurse if we are to develop meaningful theories and new knowledge to guide the expanding horizons of our practice and our persons. At the present time, we must, with flexible minds and with flexible spirits, reach for horizons that have no boundaries and limitations like those we have been forced to live with in the past.

Breaking away from old ideas and old conceptual frameworks is not an easy task at all. The leap into what may be new and unfamiliar territory is in fact quite frightening however exciting it may be to our senses and to our intellect. But this leap is necessary since the leap itself constitutes the act of creativity. And, creativity is precisely what it will take to break out of the boundaries and limitations constraining our profession and its growth in the past. In your experience of change, expansion, and growth in nursing and in your person, learn quickly how to become creative in giving shape and form to your life and to your role as a professional nurse.

As you respond to changing horizons of knowledge and attempt to live your life in a creative fashion, many obstacles will be placed in the path of your growth. To forewarn you of what you will face in the world of work, let me share with you a quote from a letter I recently received from a young graduate nurse. She wrote,

I am young relatively apolitical, and certainly naive in many respects—yet I can perceive the disparity that exists in society, in
health care, in the power structures of both! . . . change is imperative, and . . . I must be a part of such change. I am overwhelmed by
the task, frustrated by my own powerlessness and the ignorance and
apathy of my peers. I have been a practitioner for just under
5 months now, and though I suffer from reality shock . . . I can objectively identify the inherent problems in the (health care) system—no collective bargaining for nurses, incompetent nurses in
supervisory positions . . . the research disease orientation of the
physicians. While I'm struggling to establish a professional self
identity, the system sees me as a licensed worker. This question of
the dual role as professional and employee is a new one for me—
one that I must explore. While it is easy to be cynical, I am trying
not to be.[8]

This young graduate is not as naive as she thinks she is. She is most
astute about the situation she finds herself facing. She is facing un-
reasonable boundaries, boundaries limiting to her powers of thought
and action. She is facing obstacles in the path of her growth which may
well stifle that growth to the point of no growth, unless she can begin
to creatively shape her own growth in a system that will not help her
grow freely. This modern, young, university educated nurse is facing
prejudice and discriminatory practices directed toward her as a professional person. She will not escape the outcomes of our long history
of oppression as nurses and as women. You too will face what she is
facing and will need to take courageous and creative action to overcome it all, if you are not to die while still alive.

This young graduate comments upon her feelings of powerlessness
and the feeling of frustration that accompanies this state of mind and
being. You too will face these feelings of powerlessness and frustration. In the hopes of helping you deal effectively with these feelings,
let me comment briefly upon who we are as human beings. We are social beings. We are political beings. We are psychological beings with
an inner spiritual life and a cognitive style uniquely our own.

Since we as individuals are social beings, we can view ourselves as
beings constantly in motion at one sort of activity or another. We are

either relating to family, friends, colleagues, or to clients. We are creatures of much mobility. We live in a society characterized by the mobility of its people. We also live in a society where the game of power is constantly being played. This game of power is politics and politics touches every move we make as social beings. Developing ourselves as political beings determines who we are, what we do, and how far we can grow as free persons in a free society.

In view of our mobility as social and political beings, I like to think of individuals as tiny units of energy enclosed in physical bodies, and indeed that is what we are. Because of the energy contained within us, we are personal powerhouses, so to speak. Our personal energy and our personal power enables us to act or not to act, to get involved with life or to stay uninvolved. Once we become conscious of who we are as beings, we can direct our energies however we wish. In the effective use of power, we can choose to use our energies in constructive ways or we can choose to use our energies to close ourselves off from he force of life or the force of changing ideas. Energy is power. And, the effective use of energy is the key to the effective use of power.

By conceptualizing individuals as units of energy and as units of power, we can go a step further: we can think in terms of pooling this energy and in terms of pooling this power. To join an organization or to join a group is an act of pooling energies to increase our collective power to effect changes in social and political domains. The single person alone cannot do the work of a society. This takes organizations and this takes groups. Political and social action derives from the leadership of individuals and from the pooled actions of groups and organizations. It is through the interaction of individuals and groups that change of any sort is accomplished.

The effective use of your energy or power requires making the proper connections. You must move around making contacts and connections with the right people, people who will help you grow and make progress in developing your potentials and your talents. As you make the proper connections, your lives can become expanded in their horizons and in their productivity.

Finally, and perhaps most important of all, the effective use of power requires that you stay closely in touch with your inner life, growing to love who you are as a person and growing to love the talents you, and you alone, were born to develop in the course of your lifetime. Your psychological health as a self is something you must cultivate carefully as an ongoing process. The blossoming of your flower of personhood depends upon your getting intimately acquainted with the self underneath your skin, the self within your mind, within your soul. The blossoming of your self requires making distinctions between that self and the self of others you will encounter during your lifetime.

If you develop all sides of your being, you will not come down with the sickness of boredom; you will not be stifled or stopped by prejudice or discrimination; and, you can reach for emerging horizons without fear of losing your humanity. Your commencement is a timely commencement. It is a good time to be a woman. It is a good time to be a nurse. For the first time in the history of mankind, women are becoming responsible adults. And, for the first time in history of this nation, nurses are finding their voice and demanding the freedom to do their work of nursing. For the first time, nurses want and are actively seeking the powers and the opportunities to develop their talents for the good of self and for the good of society.

In closing this address, let me leave you with a bit of poetic verse you can recall when times get rough and the way gets hard as you face the inevitable prejudice that awaits you. The name of this verse is *A Place in the Sun.*

A Place in the Sun

by Jo Ann Ashley

O give us nurses a place in the sun
Where it is warm.
The rays of the sun know no
    prejudice.
The rays of the sun do not
    discriminate.
They shine on all alike.

Rainbows exist for all to see.
Why must anyone be denied the view
Of what nature has decreed a virtuous
Sight,
Free to all who will look,
Free to all who will see?

Some wish to hoard the rays of the
Sun.
Some wish to hide rainbows away for
The gaze of only a selected few.
O physicians, hospital administrators,
Medics, and emergency techs,
A place in the sun does not belong
Only to you,
It belongs to us nurses too.

Though we are women, a place in the
    sun
Belongs to us.
The sun is rightfully ours as much as
    it
Is yours.
We want our equal share.
Release us from your imposed
    limitations.
Open wide the boundaries
    surrounding us.
We want fairness and just treatment
    for
Nurses to come.

A place in the sun, we nurses will
    seek.
Our profession must be free.
Society needs the rays of our care,
No less than people need to see and
    feel
The warmth of a beaming sunbeam.

References

1. Hampshire, S. (1977, March). The future of knowledge. *The New York Review of Books* (24–5), p.18.
2. *Ibid.*
3. May, R. (1975). *The courage to create* (p. 54) New York: W. W. Norton.
4. Stavrianos, L. S. (1976). *The promise of the coming dark age* (p. 6). San Francisco: W. H. Freeman.
5. *Ibid*, p.7.
6. Barzun, J., & Graff, H. F. (1970). *The modern researcher* (p. 55) New York: Harcourt, Brace & World.
7. Arendt, H. (1959). *The human condition* (p. 170). New York: Doubleday.
8. Letter from Helen Archer to Jo Ann Ashley, December 8, 1976.

Chapter 14

REFLECTIONS ON MYTHS AND SYMBOLS PINNING NURSING DOWN*

*J*ust a brief message to the audience: I really wish to address my comments to graduating members and I hope family members, friends, and onlookers from the faculty will not be too terribly bored while I am doing so.

Also, for the information of the graduates, I bought this robe I am wearing just for this occasion. I have never worn it before and may never wear it again. So if I look a little odd to you, I want you to know I am feeling a little odd, too. However, since I am speaking to you on symbols and knew that you would be wearing yours, I wanted to wear symbolic dress also.

First, before I begin, I want to paraphrase Dory Previn by saying, if I fail to say what you want to hear, please don't put me down. I promise to tell you no lies about the profession you are entering. And what I say may have meaning for you in the future, if not now.

THE RIGHT OF PASSAGE

Traditionally, ceremonial observance of the rites of passage from one role or status to another has constituted an important occasion for

* Paper presented at the pinning ceremony, class of 1975, School of Nursing, Northern Illinois University, Carl Sandburg Auditorium, Dekalb, IL, April 20, 1975.

honored participants. Usually ritual, symbols, and myths are all a part of such rites, since it is these which give rise to ceremonies such as this pinning for you today. Pinning ceremonies have a long history in nursing and involve many of our symbols. Thus, the title of my paper, "Reflections on Myths and Symbols Pinning Nursing Down."

Since I am going to engage in a bit of reflective thinking, I'll do so by sharing with you some of the feelings I had at my own pinning ceremony. My classmates and I had earned the right to wear the white uniform and cap, signifying our graduate status. We had earned the right to have the candles on our small lamps lighted and the right to say, in unison, the Nightingale Pledge (which we did under oath with our lamps lighted). To say the least for me at that time, it was an awe-inspiring occasion. Our speaker was a physician, as was the custom at that hospital school; another custom was that of giving graduates, along with their pins, a small Merck Manual. Having completed three years of hard work, with our pins, our Merck Manuals and in stiff, starched uniforms and white shoes, we were sent out into the world of nursing work.

At my pinning ceremony, I had feelings of excitement, dedication to duty, along with some sense of humility and nervousness, since I can remember my palms sweating and my lamp shaking a bit. Both my classmates and I probably all thought that the light on our candle would go out right in the middle of saying the Nightingale Pledge. Had this happened, it would surely have been a bad omen for our future in nursing. However, though many lights did flicker, our candles burned as long as they were supposed to that night.

Although the meaning of that night was drastically changed for me, I felt inspired then. I wanted to touch the fevered brows of the sick and to bring them comfort. I wanted to heal the wounded and help the lame to walk again. Though having high aspirations, I was a bit naive back in those days and didn't think much about my place in the world as a nurse. My life and work did not change much after that pinning ceremony. In the world of work, I only did more of what I had done as a student, and was paid a meager wage for it. From that right of passage, I passed into the role of evening charge nurse on a medical-surgical unit where I had little time to touch brows. Certainly, I healed few wounds and as for the lame I cared for in those days, they are probably still not walking today.

By sharing these thoughts and reflections with you, the main point I wish to make is that if my growth had stopped with that pinning ceremony, and if I had continued to believe in the symbols and myths I believed in then, I'd be intellectually blind today, living by illusions that could not help me, my patients, or other nurses grow in professional practice, acquiring knowledge so necessary in nursing.

The Meaning of Symbols and Myths

Historically, the symbols and myths surrounding the nursing profession have given rise to illusions which all of us must seriously question today. Myths and accompanying realities influencing nursing's development have been grossly discriminatory to women in the profession and these myths and symbols should have received a more critical examination long ago. Myths give meaning to our lives. And as the times change, our myths must also change. Those no longer useful in achieving healthy development should be discarded and new ones created. This has not been the case in nursing. The task remains for us (you and me) to do this now and in the future.

I want to explore with you some of the meanings and symbols surrounding pinning ceremonies. To get at symbolic or mythical thinking, let us first look concretely at the meaning of significant words. Let us take the word pin, for example. What is a pin, that it can hold such symbolic meaning that all young nurses for a period of a century have wanted one—each wanting their school's distinctive pin? A pin is indeed a symbol in nursing, but a pin to define one is "a piece of wire for attaching something" to one's clothing or hair or a second definition, taken from Webster's dictionary, says that a pin "is a thing of small value"; it is a "trifle."

Now that we know what the non-symbolic meaning of a pin is, let me move on to define what pinning itself means. A pinning means "to fasten, join, secure, transfix, by or with a pin"; it means "to seize and hold fast." A pinning also means to "impale" and impale means to "torture or punish by fixing on a sharp stake"; to impale is "to pierce with or as with a pale." And a pale is a "stake; a pointed slat for fencing." A pale is also a "territory or district within certain bounds"; it is an enclosure implying "limits" and "bounds," as in a "cloister's pale." So says Webster.

By chasing down and analyzing the meaning of a pin and a pinning, one can get to the real root meanings of a pinning ceremony. Historically in nursing, the custom, in many schools, was that of having a physician come to speak to the nurses, honoring them with his presence. Isabel M. Stewart, a noted nurse educator, once said that the presence of the physicians was not really necessary or required at pinning ceremonies, since they all said the same thing year after year. She went on to suggest, all that was needed was a tape-recorder; if you taped one you could hear the message of all of them. Her humorous criticism of physicians was quite correct, however. They usually told nurses that they were in an honorable and dignified profession for women; they warned nurses that they could do much harm to patients if they did not remain loyal to physicians; they told them that their limited function was that of touching fevered brows and remaining cheerful however hard and tedious their work. At their pinning ceremonies, from the first decade on, nurses were told that knowledge on their part was not necessary, but beyond the limits and bounds of their sphere of functioning and thought—and, of course, a pinning, as we have seen by definition, means just this—the setting of limits and bounds beyond which a nurse is not to go; a pinning really connotes a confining and punitive affair.

To quote one physician, he told nurses that "a little knowledge was a dangerous thing, but in nursing knowledge could be fatal." After reading this in some historical papers, I wondered what ever became of those young nurses. Did they take the words of this man seriously or did they question its logic? For the myth that knowledge was dangerous for women to have was itself illogical. Myths are often illogical and are to be continuously questioned.

To repeat, a pinning means to enclose or fence in. And, historically, the nursing profession has been pinned into a subservient role under the medical profession, just because of the myths and symbols about women's intellectual and professional inferiority in comparison to men. Nursing has literally been pinned down legally and educationally. As a result, our knowledge base for practice is only now beginning to grow. Our lack of progress has been a reality because knowledge was considered to be beyond the limits and bounds of women. Nurses have been pinned to the menial role of serving others, not free to create knowledge in their own field of practice. Early nursing leaders (at least some of them) used to dream of the day when nurses would wear, along with other professionals, academic robes symbolizing their acquisition of knowledge. This was a dream in the days when colleges and universities would not admit nurses. It seems somehow ironic that now, even though we are in colleges and universities, we are still observing pinning ceremonies all over the country. Not only is it ironic, it illustrates the survival of symbolic meanings that refuse to die at any rapid rate.

There are other symbols we need to look at, so let us take the white cap and uniform. White means, "free from spot or blemish, hence, innocent or pure." Both the white uniform and the white cap symbolize purity and innocence on the part of nurses, with the cap especially representing dignity (one does have to stand rather tall and straight to keep a cap on her head and in some cases a cap can be hazardous to patient care as a result). Moreover, men in nursing do not wear them, only women. Women always have because their outward dress has symbolized dignity, purity, and innocence. Nurses have cared for the sick for a century with dedication and devotion, scarcely questioning the myths perpetuating their low social status in the professional world and in society. Only now is Kristine Hall, a Chicago nurse, questioning discriminatory dress codes in a course of law. Fired for not wearing her cap, she is the first ever to legally question this symbol.

We are probably the only professional group in society in which practitioners are forced to wear a uniform religiously. Our white uniform is a symbol saying nothing about the quality of thinking a nurse puts into her work. To get back to the meaning of words, uniform means, "having always the same form and manner as another;" it means "not varying or variable;" it means "conforming to one rule or mode" of behavior. Uniform means "presenting an undiversified appearance of surface, pattern, or conduct. It means being "consistent in conduct and in opinion."

A uniform is dress worn by persons in the same service, such as a soldier in the army, waitresses, dietitians, toilet attendants, and of course, nurses. I want you to think for yourself about the symbolic and real meaning of the nurse's uniform and decide what its meaning is in relation to professional performance.

In reality, nurses have, in a uniform manner, conformed to rules fairly consistently and uniformly all over the country. Historically, if you study what went on in one school of nursing you could know pretty well what was going on in others; practices and rules were almost the same. Uniformed nurses looked similar in outward appearance and also their inward thoughts tended to be alike because of the indoctrination in the educational system and the stereotypes held by the larger society. We have, as a result remained, for the most part, a faceless majority in the health field, operating in an isolated culture of oppressed silence.

Mythological symbols in nursing blinded young women to the truth of realities in our profession. Our use of white as a symbol representing purity, innocence, and dignity were deceptive. While nurses were taught that they belong to "an honorable profession," the whole of society would not accord them this status, or provide the donations and support needed to enable them to understand the deception in myths that bound them to roles in which they were not free to be first-class professionals, with privileges equal to men. The symbols of white cap, shoes, and dress attracted women into nursing, but such symbols illustrate the manner in which myths can become deceptive and oppressive if they are not constantly examined and modified. Our repressive symbols have not been analyzed from a historical point of view and we know few of the truths about our roots. Walking many miles in our white shoes, we were cast in the role of beasts of burden, or at the least, as sheep, unaware that we were being deceived. The lamps we supposedly carried did not light our way to insight, nor did the oath we took guide us to truth and what was for us a right as professionals.[1] It is time now that we take our symbols and myths more seriously and question them carefully.

As humans, we need our myths and symbols. We have the unique ability to invest in symbols because of the meaning they give to our lives. A piece of wire, a piece of metal, or a stone, can arouse deep emotions and feelings within us. Let us make certain that in the future our symbols do not oppress us and stifle our growth and productivity.

Since poetic language and thought provide an excellent avenue for expressing symbolic meaning, I want to share the poem on pages 260–261 with you.

It is now time for all nurses, those being pinned today and those who have been pinned for years, to question the myths and symbols pinning nursing down. The time is ripe for us to cultivate a climate in which we can all grow, a climate that will give rise to the provision of our freedom to give good nursing care to all humans who need and seek it.

REFERENCE

1. Ashley, J. A. (1975, March). *Myths and realities of prenticeship in nursing: Paternalism in practice.* (Unpublished research paper presented at the Thirteenth Annual Stewart Research Conference in Nursing.) New York: Teachers College, Columbia University.

If You Must Be Pinned

If you must be pinned
Let it be
To nothing but
The personal cost
And burden
Of gaining knowledge
To set your mind
And spirit free.

Knowledge does not rise
From the creations of
The innocent or the
Pure.
For the paths of knowledge
Are often dim and dark,
Leading one into
The blackness of the
Unknown.

For all to eventually
Know the meaning
Of truth
Some must take
This route,
Beyond the bounds of
Conformity and security,
Though it leaves them
Less than innocent,
Less than pure.

If you want to be
Enlightened
Seek not to remain
Innocent,
But to awaken your mind
To truths that are not
Always pure.

Trust no other
Mind
As much as your own.
Seek no comfort
That does not have
Its base within,
Remembering still that
In the realm of
Knowledge
There are no rules,
Only guidelines
That change with
Each forward step
You take.

Meaning itself, you see,
Is a myth,
And without knowledge
It does not exist.
If you must be pinned,
You will make no mistake
If you drive your own stake.
Then you can move it,
Shift it,
Alter its position,
And thus extend the
Bounds and limits of
Your territory
As you see fit.

Let pinning be for you
A symbol
For defining your
Own boundaries, limits,
And grooves.

Pin yourself to
A search
For knowledge
And you will
Find your own myths
That hold meaning
For you.

In your mind's eye
Transpose your
Uniforms
Into academic robes,
You are not alike,
But unique.
And free,
Having talents and taste
That differ
From those who sit
Close to you.

Your thoughts are not
The same as your neighbor's
Thoughts.
Nor your dreams the same
As their dreams.
Keep this in mind
And do not remain
Uniformed
For that will never
Set you free.

Conform if you must,
But do not

Let the hinges on
Your pin rust,
Or you will find
Yourself
In a rut,
Speaking what your
Neighbor speaks,
Seeking what your
Neighbor seeks,
Though it may leave
You less than
Free.

Do search and research,
And count the cost of
Where you place your
Stakes,
To be fenced in and
Enclosed is not a
Very worthy goal.

If you must be pinned,
Know when,
Know where,
Know why.
This do and
Your human spirit
And intellectual potential
Will not die
With years that fly.

Index

610.73   JoAnn Ashley.
JOA

$32.50

DATE			

BAKER & TAYLOR